The Body in History, Culture, and the Arts

The aim of this book is to explore the body in various historical contexts and to take it as a point of departure for broader historiographical projects. The chapters in the volume present the ways in which the body constitutes a valuable and productive object of historical analysis, especially as a lens through which to trace histories of social, political, and cultural phenomena and processes. More specifically, the authors use the body as a tool for critical reexamination of particular histories of human experience and of societal and cultural practices, thus contributing to the burgeoning area of body history in terms of both specific case studies as well as historiography in general.

Justyna Jajszczok is an Assistant Professor at the Institute of English, University of Silesia, Katowice, Poland.

Aleksandra Musiał is an Assistant Professor at the Institute of English Cultures and Literatures, University of Silesia, Katowice, Poland.

Routledge Studies in Cultural History

The Transatlantic Genealogy of American Anglo-Saxonism
Michael Modarelli

Anxieties of Belonging in Settler Colonialism
Australia, Race and Place
Lisa Slater

Families, Values, and the Transfer of Knowledge in Northern Societies, 1500–2000
Edited by Ulla Aatsinki, Johanna Annola, and Mervi Kaarninen

A History of Euphoria
The Perception and Misperception of Health and Well-Being
Christopher Milnes

The History of the Vespa
An Italian Miracle
Andrea Rapini

Children and Globalization
Multidisciplinary Perspectives
Edited by Hoda Mahmoudi and Steven Mintz

A History of Shaolin
Buddhism, Kung Fu and Identity
Lu Zhouxiang

Heroism as a Global Phenomenon in Contemporary Culture
Edited by Barbara Korte, Simon Wendt and Nicole Falkenhayner

The Body in History, Culture, and the Arts
Edited by Justyna Jajszczok and Aleksandra Musiał

For more information about this series, please visit: www.routledge.com/Routledge-Studies-in-Cultural-History/book-series/SE0367

The Body in History, Culture, and the Arts

Edited by Justyna Jajszczok
and Aleksandra Musiał

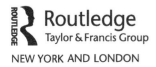

Routledge
Taylor & Francis Group

NEW YORK AND LONDON

First published 2019
by Routledge
52 Vanderbilt Avenue, New York, NY 10017

and by Routledge
2 Park Square, Milton Park, Abingdon, Oxon, OX14 4RN

First issued in paperback 2020

Routledge is an imprint of the Taylor & Francis Group, an informa business

Library of Congress Cataloging-in-Publication Data
A catalog record for this title has been requested

ISBN 13: 978-0-367-67124-2 (pbk)
ISBN 13: 978-0-367-20955-1 (hbk)

Typeset in Sabon
by Apex CoVantage, LLC

Contents

Figures

Introduction

"The Past Is Written on My Body": Bodies and History

Justyna Jajszczok and Aleksandra Musiał

It is no easy task to write an adequate introduction to a collection of essays that undertake to consider the body at intersections with history in such a disparate array of periods, contexts, and even methods. But while an account of the body in history that would totalize the ways in which the issue might be approached remains elusive, an endeavor such as this volume is not necessarily hopeless as a cohesive project. Evidently, the body remains "productive as a category of historical analysis" (Blayney, in this volume), as testified to by the breadth of subjects analyzed and discussed in this book: the variety itself illustrates how useful the body proves as an avenue into a better understanding of history. This entanglement of the human body with the past—in so many ways *its* past, after all—is of course not surprising since, as Donna McCormack put it, "[f]lesh is woven into history as both the bloody deaths necessary to achieve the desired goals and the skin on which it has become possible to write these new foundational narratives" (2014, 2).

Indeed, the body, historically contextualized, has been studied in relation to a whole range of disciplines and approaches. To mention only some of the more recent cases, following the pioneering works that tended to focus on bodies in given historical periods such as the Renaissance or Early Modernity, some recent transhistorical studies have focused on the relationship between the body and more narrowly defined areas of critical inquiry, such as the history of human sexuality (Toulalan and Fisher 2013) or the history of disability and impairment (Mounsey and Booth 2016). Another trend has been to provide "organ-by-organ" histories, which look at the human body as a unit whose particular history—or histories of its component parts—may be traced, especially in the context of medical and scientific history (Alberti 2016; Aldersey-Williams 2013). There has also been interest in examining continuity and change in bodily practices and in attitudes toward the body across history but in a defined geographical/cultural location, either in Europe from prehistory to now (Robb and Harris 2013) or in the contemporary West as opposed to its past (Alberti 2016).

This volume takes a less focalized approach as a whole, and instead, by the juxtaposition of its parts and chapters, reveals the variously conceptualized body as a fundamental category of historical study, its peculiar but indelible significance stemming out of its somewhat dual nature. The first aspect of this duality may be illustrated by the observation that the body turns out to function as a potent and ubiquitous metaphor. Since it is the most immediate apparatus through which we can observe and interact with the outside world, our perception of reality is inextricably filtered through our bodies. It is no surprise, then, that our own sense of the body so often becomes a form of language used to translate, or perhaps even metaphorically tame, elements of the external world. Consider the two great unknowns of human exploration: space and oceans. Both are beyond human reach, one too distant, the other too deep; both are immense and still largely undiscovered, perhaps even unknowable; both, by the virtue of their sheer scale, are putting human beings in their right place, insignificant specks in the grander scheme of things. Perhaps this is the reason why we use the metaphor of the body when describing and explaining the universe: to rhetorically reduce the universe to a manageable concept that may be easier to accept and understand. And so "celestial bodies" and "bodies of water" bring to mind large quantities and vast expanses but, through their corporeal associations, can also inspire familiarity and affinity.

If we continue this line of inquiry into the body's thrust into the realm of metaphor, we will also find that in history the metaphor bleeds dangerously into the (corpo)real, from history as discipline to history as past: the corpus of texts, the body of history, always conceals within it masses of bodies, people physically embedded in their realities as they unfolded in time, experiencing the outside world as pleasure or pain. It is the body, again, that allows us access to those bygone realities as they were lived through and felt.

An example will illustrate this. In 413 BC, the ill-fated Athenian expedition to subdue Sicily ended in utter defeat and disaster. As we know from Thucydides (7.86), the authorities of Syracuse, the most powerful Sicilian settlement, then imprisoned the Athenian soldiers whom they had taken prisoner in the city's stone quarries. A great deal of suffering was endured in the following eight months: "at least 7,000" hostages, the historian tells us,

> were crowded together in a narrow pit, where, since there was no roof over their heads, they suffered first from the heat of the sun and the closeness of the air; and then, in contrast, came on the cold autumnal nights, and the change in temperature brought disease among them. Lack of space made it necessary for them to do everything on the same spot; and besides there were bodies all heaped together on top of one another of those who had fallen from their wounds or from the change of temperature or other such causes, so

that the smell was insupportable. At the same time they suffered from hunger and from thirst.

(7.87)

This might just be the most *human* paragraph in the *History of the Peloponnesian War*, and it is no coincidence that it arrives in the form of a catalog of bodily anguish and misery. Thucydides' resolute detachment and missionary objectivity dictate his cool, crisp style; but the reader, who might otherwise remain unmoved by the stories of the Greeks told by the historian, or who might find their motivations, customs, culture, and even psychology bizarre or alien, will recognize immediately a human familiarity with the Athenians imprisoned in the quarry. Even if notions such as sympathy for the defeated or concern for human rights might well be said to be conditioned by one's culture, this is not the case in the stripped-down matter of physical suffering, of what a human body *feels*; we all bleed, and we are all united in what makes our bodies suffer. Most simply put—and at the very least—no one would want to experience for *themselves* what those long gone Athenians underwent.

It is because of this basic affinity—perhaps the basic substance of the human condition—that the human body, when considered in the context of its historical and cultural (social, political, spiritual, etc.) entanglements, can never be simply an end product of discourse. As one scholar of the body observed, "we are tied to the world by our bodies" (Alberti 2016, 2), and so the body's own materiality always pulls it down toward the empirical, the *lived through* and *felt*.

The body, therefore, can be considered in the context of this duality. On the one hand, it is a "total metaphor," performing something of a vertical conquest of experience through language, its symbolic ubiquity speaking to its role as an agent of the physical reality. But, on the other hand (here is the metaphor again!), the body is also the "total state of being," our anchorage to here and now, and, perhaps most importantly from the point of view of this volume, a method of accessing experiences in the past. Chris Mounsey captures this notion when he writes that "[t]he language of the body, the body of you or of me, or of any character in any piece of literature is the same language because it terminates upon the body and articulates it, albeit that the body in each case is different. But it must be remembered that each body is the 'same only different' from every other" (2016, 2–3). This totality of the body is what allows us to better connect to the experiences of people in the past.

The "sameness but difference" of human bodies, especially as it pertains to understanding history, requires some elaboration. In the monumental *The Body in History*, the editors point out that

[t]o understand the body . . . it is essential to set it in its own cultural, social, political and material frame of reference. In turn, this

frame of reference has to be understood as *historical*. . . . The body is not a universally shared physical object whose historical continuity comes from its unchanging biological structure, but rather something emergent through history. The body is in history; indeed, the body *is* history.

(Robb and Harris 2013, 4; emphasis in original)

If this is true—the body *is* history—then history itself should be understood as something that emerges through the body.

In other words, here we arrive at yet another metaphor, this one of the snake eating its own tail: there is no history without the body, but to study the body, the contexts that embed it must first be considered. It is possible that the body must always remain elusive in this way, at once a unifying phenomenon of human experience and one that escapes universalization, or indeed loses its epistemological potential when reduced to a simple abstraction. Thus, in addition to providing us with the sense of a basic human affinity that strengthens an empathetic approach to historical periods, the body also constitutes an access point to the past in that, through studying bodies both at precise moments and across time, we might better study history itself. So perhaps this is what we must always do: look to the specific body, entangled in a specific moment in history, and try to better understand the moment by better understanding the body.

The chapters in this volume speak to this special position of the human body. The authors engage it as both subject and object of history and as embedded in definite, historicized social realities. No other approach is viable, of course, since in the middle of a map of concepts, such as sex, gender, race, health, and hygiene, is the body with which all of these are inextricably involved. Part of the reason why "the body *is* history," that history emerges through it, is that the human body in a social context is always involved in a process of creating and defying its own binary oppositions: sexualized vs. sexless bodies, exoticized vs. normalized bodies, dirty and diseased bodies vs. clean and godly bodies.

To provide an example, the tensions between these categories were particularly apparent in Victorian times when body-centered issues came to the forefront. As Sean Purchase asserts, "[s]ocially and politically, the Victorians took issue with the body on a number of levels, particularly the woman's body" (2006, 12). He goes on to divide the nineteenth-century discussion regarding the corporeal into two streams, both of which functioned as a means and tool of othering nonstandard bodies. On the one hand, there was the body of a prostitute, attitudes to which were demonstrated through the infamous Contagious Diseases Acts of the 1860s: an act in effect legitimizing state rape under the dubious cover of protection against venereal diseases (Luddy 2013, 415–419). On the other hand, classifying and identifying the body as a dangerous tool of destroying societal order was the one propagated by beliefs stemming from criminal anthropology of Cesare Lombroso and Max Nordau's degeneration theories (Purchase 2006, 12–13).

Here, then, we see the body and history exerting mutual influence on each other: while bodies, as objects of discourses, shape policy and societal attitudes, they are also subject to the effects of these. But more can be gained from an analysis of a historical period and its cultural milieu through the body. To stay for a moment with the Victorians, the body as the source of social destruction was also a fascinating topic for the newly emerging popular literature of the urban or imperial gothic genre of the time. The internally and symbolically divided body of Dr. Jekyll, the aesthetically and morally suspended body of Dorian Gray, the hideously misshapen and misgendered body of *The Beetle*'s antagonist: all of them speak of the powers bodies hold and exert, within the confines of their narratives, and outside them. Literal bodies, paradoxically, are presented as anchors, keeping their owners within the bounds of reality, and as a means of escaping those same bounds. Before Freud's unconscious, the Victorians could read and see the bodies on social display as manifestations of basic drives.

Moreover, this rising interest in processes, mechanics, and behaviors expressed through the human body could be traced to the population boom cities experienced in the nineteenth century. The concentration of people in all areas of life seemed as inconvenient as inevitable. Kathryn Hughes describes it in particularly colorful words: "Strangers who would never previously have set eyes on one another increasingly found themselves in an involuntarily intimate embrace at the factory bench, the railway station, the lodging house, the beach or on the top deck of an omnibus. Other people's sneezes, bums, elbows, smells, snores, farts and breathy whistles were, quite literally, in your face" (2017, xi). These impressions seem very familiar to us today, with our experiences of limited personal space on crowded buses and trains. Yet, our constant exposure to other people's bodies in a way desensitizes us to their presence, their corporeality brought to us only in moments of broken societal norms: public urination, spitting, vomiting, or public breastfeeding (whose presumed controversiality speaks, of course, to the structures of power and politics of representation current in the society we are living in rather than to the act itself possessing any transgressive quality).

This points to the validity of the distinction that could be traced to the Victorians: of female bodies politicized by ideologically dictated norms and standards and of pathologized bodies reduced to their functions and processes as viewed by medical sciences. In very general terms, the chapters within this volume follow the same patterns of analysis of bodies at specific historical moments and across changes in time. Here meet the histories of female bodies and the histories of "pathologized" bodies— Othered, criminalized, annihilated—discussed in the collected chapters, the categories exchanging accounts of mistreatments, mishandlings, misrepresentations, and misunderstandings.

The aim of the book, then, is to explore the body in various historical contexts and to take it as a point of departure for broader historiographical projects. The chapters in the volume present the ways in which the body constitutes a valuable and productive object of historical analysis, especially as a lens through which to trace histories of social, political, and cultural phenomena and processes. More specifically, the authors use the body as a tool for critical reexamination of particular histories of human experience and of societal and cultural practices. Thus, while individual contributions to the volume focus on specific body-related histories, the overall goal of this collection it to accentuate the place, the role, and the use of the body in history and historiography.

Each chapter on its own concerns a particular historical period and body-related subject, which offers methodological, analytical, and interpretational models of studying these specific histories. On the whole, the chapters in this volume share a concern for *what* the body as studied by a historian *is*, or, in other words, for *how* to make the body an object of historiography and of historical analysis. Instead of approaching the body from a strictly material, physiological, or medical perspective— or, conversely, instead of approaching it solely as the end product of discourse—the chapters look at the collective body/actual human bodies enmeshed in society and culture as well as the practices that stem from such entanglement.

The authors in the first part of this volume ("The Liminal Body"), employing similar approaches and methodologies, present particular historical texts that focus on the body suspended in liminal spaces. William Leeming investigates the idea of *lusus naturae* (a joke of nature) as an organizing principle of Nature's *ingenio* and the "serious play" of scientific inquiry in *De Monstris*. While he draws from illustrations in Liceti's encyclopedic compilation to present the liminal bodies of monstrous human-animal hybrids, Jacqueline Susann Holler uses the example of a heterogeneous toolkit employed by a Mexican midwife to explore the notion of the birthing body as a "contact zone" at the intersection of indigenous and colonial medical practices. Holler's chapter is based on information obtained through studies of Mexican Inquisition documentations regarding witchcraft accusation cases. In a similar vein, Carlo Bovolo reviews articles published in *La Civiltà Cattolica*, an Italian Jesuit periodical, which record the discussion between medical and religious scholars debating the validity of symptoms/symbols of sainthood at the end of the nineteenth century.

In Part II ("The Modern Body"), Steffan Blayney and Christopher E. Forth consider the physical bodies of people at the beginning of the twentieth century and at the dawn of modernity. Though their particular approaches differ—Blayney rereads the history of labor at the intersection with scientific knowledge while Forth is interested in the deeper psycho-social layers of anti-fat prejudice—their conclusions overlap, offering an insight into the period's nascent preoccupation with efficiency and control over the human body, which would ensure a better, ordered world. Both chapters also point at the historical moment in question as the genesis of cultural trends that persist and become even more prominent today.

Claude Lacroix and Kylo-Patrick R. Hart, in Part III ("The Visual Body"), look at how visual representations of the body have been used to demarcate social inclusion and exclusion at specific historical moments. Where Lacroix considers the body ideals of interwar Germany promoted in opposition to the disfigured bodies of First World War veterans, symbolic of the country's defeat and decline, Hart examines the first decade of the AIDS epidemic in the US and the specific representational strategies of marking infected men as Othered and repulsive, symbolic of sinful lifestyles. Though the chapters concern two very different visual cultures and two different groups of very visible outcasts, they offer parallel analyses of the social ramifications of disgust induced by representations that equate aesthetics with morality and the acceptability of appearance with the permission to belong.

In the fourth part of the book ("The Punished Body"), Willemijn Ruberg and CalvinJohn Smiley both touch upon the issue of punishment: how bodies of criminals and convicts become disembodied, and instead stripped down to their synecdochic external signifiers. Ruberg traces how the hair, remaining the object and the end of official disciplinary measures, changes from the target of early modern criminal punishment to an isolated piece of evidence in contemporary forensics, while Smiley explores how and to what extent the US prison system impacts the body of a convict. Both explain how visibility of the punished body influences and shapes the internal narrative of people inhabiting those bodies, their identity, and place in society.

The volume's concluding fifth part ("The Entangled Body") includes chapters by Anna Kisiel and David Schauffler, both of which use the image of the body reproduced in works of art—a series of paintings and theatrical plays, respectively—to unlock meanings of historical moments and periods. Both authors are interested in a duality: the symbolic functions of the body and its historical corporeality. They both treat the body as a gatekeeper to the problems it itself poses, and they both use theory to extricate it from its entanglement in historical context, symbolism, and representation. Kisiel considers the possibility of connecting to a particular moment during the Holocaust through an artistic rendering of it captured in a photograph, while Schauffler reexamines nuances of medieval/Renaissance sovereignty embodied in the king via plays by Shakespeare. The authors thus offer two models of theorizing the body in relation to (its own) history.

Finally, it is perhaps worth pointing out that since this volume emphasizes the historical aspect of the body, the more personal and visceral relation to the body may seem pushed to the margin—but this is not the case. Roxane Gay begins her memoir with a simple sentence: "Every body has a story and a history" (2017, 1); and thus, in this short but powerful statement, she brings together the notions of a body caught in history and a body inhabited by a person. Indeed, the historically suspended bodies our contributors write about all tell stories of singular bodies whose experiences and memories are indispensable in allowing their history to be told. Gay's story, told with almost uncomfortable candor, is a story of a body divided into the past, with its experiences and traumas, and the present, in which the physical and mental manifestations of the suffering are displayed. "The past," she writes, "is written on my body" (2017, 37).

Gay concludes on an assertive note: "In writing this memoir of my body, in telling you these truths about my body, I am sharing my truth and mine alone" (2017, 277). Having traced the history of the body lost and regained, broken and mended, Gay reiterates the truth that should always be at the back of our minds: the body is a place, a tool, and an experience. It collectively tells a story of all of us and, individually, of every single one of us. No*body* can escape their body; every body has a story.

References

Alberti, Fay Bound. 2016. *This Mortal Coil: The Human Body in History and Culture*. New York: Oxford University Press.

Aldersey-Williams, Hugh. 2013. *Anatomies: A Cultural History of the Human Body*. New York: W. W. Norton & Company.

Gay, Roxane. 2017. *Hunger: A Memoir of (My) Body*. London: Corsair.

Hughes, Kathryn. 2017. *Victorians Undone: Tales of Flesh in the Age of Decorum*. London: 4th Estate.

Luddy, Maria. 2013. "Prostitution from 1800." In *The Routledge History of Sex and the Body*, edited by Sarah Toulalan and Kate Fisher, 409–426. London: Routledge.

McCormack, Donna. 2014. *Queer Postcolonial Narratives and the Ethics of Witnessing*. New York: Bloomsbury.

Mounsey, Chris. 2016. "Introduction: Speaking Forwards in History." In *The Variable Body in History*, edited by Chris Mounsey and Stan Booth, 1–11. Oxford: Peter Lang.

Mounsey, Chris, and Stan Booth, eds. 2016. *The Variable Body in History*. Oxford: Peter Lang.

Purchase, Sean. 2006. *Key Concepts in Victorian Literature*. Basingstoke: Palgrave.

Robb, John, and Oliver J. T. Harris, eds. 2013. *The Body in History: Europe from the Paleolithic to the Future*. New York: Cambridge University Press.

Thucydides. 1972. *History of the Peloponnesian War*. Revised edition. Translated by Rex Warner. London: Penguin Books.

Toulalan, Sarah, and Kate Fisher, eds. 2013. *The Routledge History of Sex and the Body: 1500 to the Present*. London: Routledge.

Part I
The Liminal Body

1 Fortunio Liceti's Strategic Use of *Lusus Naturae* in *De Monstris* (1634–1665) and the Self-Assured Semiology of Naturalized Early Modern Science

William Leeming

Introduction

Anne Blair (2003) has drawn attention to an immense surge in the printing of encyclopedic compilations between 1550 and 1700 in Europe that amounted to, in her words, an "information overload." She indicates that, by the end of the sixteenth century, there was a widely held belief that there were too many books in the world for any single scholar to read and remain well-informed of *all* available knowledge. This fueled "the production of many more books, often especially large ones, designed to remedy the problem—from new genres like the universal bibliography and the book review to new (or not-so-new) contributions to well-established genres, including the florilegium, the dictionary, and the encyclopedic compilation" (Blair 2003, 12). At the same time, as Brian Ogilvie (2003, 2008) has shown, pre-Linnaean approaches to sorting and arranging the knowledge found in the almanacs, chronicles, and encyclopedic compilations of the period bore little resemblance to a taxonomic science in the modern-day sense. Indeed, in the context of the encyclopedic compilations on monsters, authors and publishers often trawled ancient annals, medieval chronicles, travelers' reports, and other documentary sources in a random and haphazard manner. Rudolf Wittkower went so far as to complain that "the sober and scientific approach was often overshadowed by the indiscriminate discussion of the available 'cases': mythological creatures, imaginary monsters and general descriptions in literature were allowed to rank on the same level as direct observations, and a number of standard illustrations were repeated in scores of books for more than a century to represent different monsters" (1942, 46).

Among the earliest of the encyclopedic compilations on monsters was Jakob Rueff's *Trostbüchle* of 1554 which, in Germany, was followed soon thereafter by the *Wunderzeichen* of Job Fincel in 1556 and Conrad Lycosthenes' *Wunderwerck* in 1557. Other well-known German encyclopedic compilations appeared in the seventeenth century by Christoph

Irenäus, Andreas Engel, Johannes Wolf, and Johannes Prätorius. Similar encyclopedic approaches were taken in France, notably the *Histoires prodigieuses* of Pierre Boaistuau (1560) and *Des monstres tant terrestres que marins, avec leurs portraits* of Ambroise Paré (1573). Compilations were also beginning to appear in Italy at that time, including Fortunio Liceti's *De Monstris*.

Fortunio Liceti (1577–1657) was a physician born in Genoa and chair of Aristotelian Philosophy at the University of Pisa before moving nine years later to the University of Padua. His *De Monstrorum Causis, Natura et Differentiis* was first published in 1616. A lavishly illustrated second edition was subsequently published in Padua in 1634, including an engraved frontispiece by Giovanni Battista Bissoni. A further edition was produced in Amsterdam in 1665 with the title *De Monstris*. The two volumes that make up *De Monstris* mostly include accounts of monsters and monstrous births selected from ancient annals, medieval chronicles, and travelers' reports. The images feature monsters in the state of nature, either standing, walking, or running in grasslands and forests. Most of the monsters are missing or have supernumerary limbs. There are numerous images of conjoined twins. A small collection of figures of the monstrous races of antiquity are interspersed among the illustrations of Book II, including blemmyes (folio131v), cyclops (folio133v), and hairy wild men (folios149v, 158r). An appendix follows with texts and illustrations taken from the work of Nicolas Tulp, the Dutch surgeon made famous in Rembrandt's *The Anatomy Lesson of Dr Nicolaes Tulp*, and Thomas Bartholin, a Danish physician, mathematician, and theologian who became famous for his anatomical studies of the lymphatic system in humans.

De Monstris is mostly celebrated in the history of science and medicine as a ground-breaking work in descriptive teratology, i.e., the study of abnormalities of embryonic development and congenital malformations as well as other forms of anomalous physiological development (Fisher 1866; Wittkower 1942; Daston and Park 1998; Bates 2001). Indeed, Isidore Geoffroy Saint-Hilaire, who coined the neologism "teratology" in the 1830s, credited Liceti as having pioneered the discipline (Lazzarini 2011, 427). Specifically, Liceti's system of two principal categories of monsters has been regarded as a crucial early example of a pre-Linnaean taxonomy for the scientific observation and clinical anatomy of teratology. But, that being said, Liceti's propensity for an ambivalent analysis of the monstrous included an investigation of what lies behind the temporal and spatial heterogeneity of monsters and what humans could expect to comprehend in terms of Nature's *ingenio*, as well as the presence of recurring forms in nature that reenact their own conditions of possibility. I focus on the latter in this chapter.

The chapter begins with background to the way Europeans approached the problems of monstrosity and monstrousness prior to the seventeenth century. There follows a brief account of the taxonomic principles of *De*

Monstris. The main focus of the chapter, however, is an investigation of what I refer to as Liceti's strategic use of *lusus naturae* (i.e., a "joke of Nature"). I argue that *lusus naturae* appears in *De Monstris* alongside the *serio ludere* (i.e., "serious play") of scientific investigation. I contend that the liminal space in which *lusus naturae* appears brings with it the potential for breaking away from colloquial understandings of the empirical presence of natural phenomena.

The Problems of Monster, Monstrosity, and Monstrousness

As Georges Canguilhem (1962) was quick to point out, historical use of the terms "monster," "monstrosity," and "monstrousness" has not been interchangeable. For Canguilhem, monstrosity is the effect produced or caused by monstrousness. And monstrousness is to be found in the act or acts believed to cause monstrosity during formal investigation and with a view to normative judgment.

The etymology of "monster" leads to the Latin *monere* and the idea of warning (Dorrian 2000, 312). Etymologically, to be a monster is to be a sign, a portent, or display. This accurately describes European accounts of monsters prior to the sixteenth century, which tended to focus exclusively on religious interpretations of what a monster prophesized (Niccoli 1990; Daston and Park 1998; Hsia 2004; Cheng 2012; Verner 2016). Monstrous births were time and again interpreted as evidence of divine providence, representing signs from God "in response to perceived lapses in moral order" (Bates 2005, 141). Indeed, early accounts of monsters and monstrous births were almost always interpreted as "signs of the wrath of God toward man and his sins, a source of deep anguish that had little to do with the 'amazement' that the other unusual wonders of creation aroused" (Cusumano 2013, 158). The allegorical figure of the monster in the sixteenth century presumed a fixed identification of what was illustrated; the problem was to assign meaning to what it was that was actually being depicted (Hampton 2004, 184). By locating the specific interpretation of the given sign, one could find its corresponding meaning in the larger chain of signs. The world could be read like a text whose words were meaningful to those properly trained in its language. For Europeans living in the period, all created things were linked together in a world of microcosms and macrocosms (Ashworth 1990).

By way of an example, in 1523 Martin Luther and Philipp Melanchthon published a pamphlet that featured two woodcuts by Lucas Cranach the Elder entitled *The Papal Ass of Rome* and *The Monk—Calf* as "reproofs of monastic and papal corruption" (Daston and Park 1998, 187) (see Figure 1.1). *The Papal Ass* exemplifies a genre of allegorized composites with its head of a donkey, scaled limbs, cloven and taloned feet, a trunk-like hand, and a womanly torso. *The Monk—Calf*, on the other hand, was reportedly based on the actual birth of a calf with a

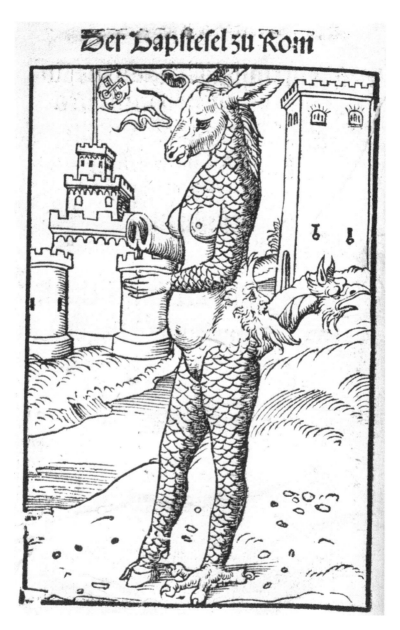

Figure 1.1 (a and b) Lucas Cranach the Elder, woodcut illustrations for Martin Luther and Philipp Melanchon, *Deuttung der Czwo Grewliche[n] Figuren Bapstesels czu Rom und Munchkalbs zu Freyberg ijnn Meysszen funden* (1523)

Image courtesy of the Bayerische Staatsbibliothek. Bayerische Staatsbibliothek München, Res/Slg.Faust 115, fol. A1 verso and recto. (CC BY-NC-SA 4.0)

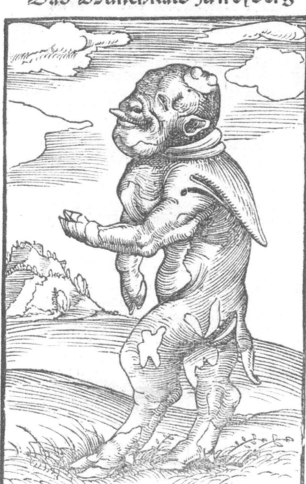

Figure 1.1 (a and b) (Continued)

cowl-like flap of flesh on its neck. Luther and Melanchthon proclaimed that the calf was a prophecy that "the monastic state was 'nothing other than a false and lying appearance and outward display of a holy, godly life'" (Daston and Park 1998, 188).

As Barbara Maria Stafford has argued, the use of analogy is "a demonstrative or evidentiary practice—putting the visible into relationship with the invisible and manifesting the effect of that momentary unison" (1999,

23–24). Analogy supports the vision of ordered relationships "articulated as similarity-in-difference" (Stafford 1999, 9). The veracity of the accounts of *The Papal Ass* and *The Monk—Calf* are to be judged by their nearness to the truth, i.e., *truthlikeness*, rather than their verifiability. The religious and political upheavals of the Protestant Reformation in the sixteenth century occasioned the use of a strategy Jerome Bruner has dubbed "coherence by contemporaneity"; that is, the "belief that things happening at the same time must be connected" (1991, 19). This was related to "connecting the lot into one coherent whole—connecting, not subsuming, not creating historical-causal entailments, but winding it into story" (1991, 20). The concept of the monster held the key to the unfolding space of signification of which experience and expectations may or may not form a part. Moreover, the monster is a prolepsis, the representation or assumption of a future act or development as if presently existing or accomplished. *As an event*, on the one hand, it is never-to-be-repeated. On the other, *as an episode of monstrousness* it represents a heterochrony (i.e., many times existing at the same time).

The understanding of what it meant to be monstrous is said to have changed by the early eighteenth century. Janvier Moscoso, for example, has written that monstrosity became naturalized in the sense of "attempts to explain away, or naturalize, the sentiment of wonder" (1998, 362). The natural world could "take on odd shapes and sometimes seem to reverse the ordering of imperfect and perfect, so that the 'prose du monde' becomes either self-referential, pointing not at something invisible and ideal but rather at itself as form" (Randall 1996, 3). What is meant to be a monster was rationalized in the eighteenth century to the extent that moral and metaphysical explanations of monstrosity were spurned in favor of what could be observed and classified (Wolfe 2005; Cusumano 2013). Even so, I will argue in what follows that the path to what was becoming naturalized and rationalized did not lead, as one might expect, to a consensus about general rules by which a given phenomenon might be included in a category of monstrousness.

The Science of *De Monstris*

As already noted, Fortunio Liceti was chair of Aristotelian Philosophy at the universities of Pisa and Padua. Suitably, his approach to theorizing reproduction, conception, and generation was closely aligned with what Aristotle had written. It is noteworthy that Aristotle offered two approaches to studying embryonic development. First, the structure (matter) of the animal is *preformed* and grows larger (*preformationism*) and, second, that structure develops progressively (*epigenesis*). At the root of the Aristotelian preformation/epigenesis dichotomy lay the division of the nature of all biological substances into their "formal nature" and their "material nature" (Henry 2006, 426–427). The salient point for purposes of studying monstrosity is that a robust theory of four causes (material, efficient, formal, and final) for scrutinizing the course of action for the transmission of characteristics from parents to offspring was vigorously worked out and incorporated into the teaching of medicine in Europe using tracts from Aristotle's *De Generatione Animalium* and *Physics* (Boylan 1984, 93–95).

The material cause affected what is to be formed and the range of all possible outcomes in embryonic development. At the point of conception, the action of the father of a child represents an efficient cause. The efficient cause is what puts the whole process in motion. But efficient cause is itself incomplete. Rather, all efficient causes are regulated by formal causes. And this is regulated by Nature. Nature provides the formal/final causes in conception. Nature "as end" brings about the organism's fully developed form (i.e., infant through to maturity or adult form) while nature "as mover" refers to the potentiality that exists *a priori* inside the developing embryo that directs the process toward its end. On the one hand, teleological activity arises from the individual's internal organic form. Form is not independent of matter. It is embodied in matter. The individual maintains its organic form by holding its end within itself. Moreover, what exists *a priori* inside the developing embryo includes inherited properties from its ancestors. This, in turn, suggests what Norman Crowe called a "timelessness within the temporal": the existence of a persistent *or* recurring structure or object that reenacts its own conditions of possibility (1997, 156). The materiality of such a substance or process is sustained across time by the tacit substitution of its parts in a manner that suggests both *metachronism* (i.e., the placing of an event after it has occurred) and *prochronism* (i.e., the placing of it before). And while the Aristotelian mind-set stressed the union of matter and form as constituting an independent entity, the substantial form of the entity represented what it has in common with its kind, what made it a member of a class of beings. In effect, an entity's distinctive features made it unique (i.e., an individual) *by accident*: "*Accidental form . . .* can change while its substantial or specific being remains unaffected. Accidental forms are perceptible; they can be analyzed in terms of the manifest properties associated with the elements. Substantial form in itself, as opposed to its effects, remains hidden from the senses" (Copenhaver 1990, 273; italics in the original).

In the sixteenth and seventeenth centuries, discussion of an entity's uniqueness became focused and nowhere more clearly than in the discussion of monsters. This involved a line of inquiry into the environmental causes of *malformation*. In the context of *De Monstris*, this meant inquiry into Nature's *ingenio* and the idea that Nature's involvement in the creation of monsters went beyond what humans *could expect to see* with respect to recurring forms that reenact their own conditions of possibility.

Nature's *Ingenio* and *Lusus Naturae*

The popular and well-known images of Cranach the Elder's *Papal Ass of Rome* and the *Monk—Calf* reappear in *De Monstris* alongside other famous prodigies including the Ravenna monster, a monster that first appeared in *Des monstres tant terrestres que marins, avec leurs portraits* of Ambroise Paré (1573). Ostensibly, Liceti's goal was to categorize the physical traits they shared in common with other manifestations of monstrosity. For example, the Ravenna monster is depicted in Book II (folio 234r) for purposes of showing what it shares with a comparable case in which a category of monster has horns. Quite simply, horns can be explained in terms of being the result of a superabundance of matter (see Figure 1.2). By comparison, the horned monsters of folio 234r are more complicated and require special attention (see Figure 1.3). On a high level of generality, then, monstrosity in *De Monstris* reflects what Victor Buchli (2010) calls "presencing."

Buchli has approached the broader question of presence as one of sensorial engagement, "all of us being co-present, physically near and visually available to us in terms of corporeal proximity to one another in

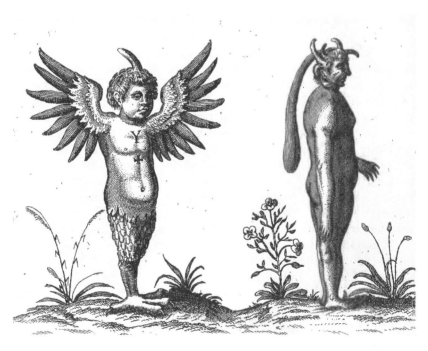

Figure 1.2 Engraving with Ravenna Monster for Book II, folio 234r, *De Monstris*
(1665). Amstelodami: Sumptibus Andreae Frisii, MDCLXV [1665]

Image courtesy of the Boston Medical Library.

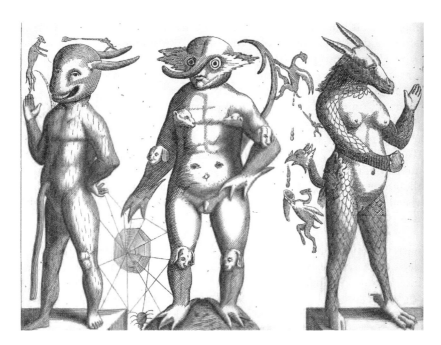

Figure 1.3 Engraving with the Krakow monster and the Papal Ass of Rome for
Book II, folio 256r, *De Monstris* (1665). Amstelodami: Sumptibus
Andreae Frisii, MDCLXV [1665]

Image courtesy of the Boston Medical Library.

the same room, village, pace, building, encampment, etc., as we might
understand it in colloquial empiricist terms" (2010, 186). Simultaneously,
Buchli maintains, there is a decidedly "unreal" register or milieu in which
other kinds of *things* are "co-present" including the "ancestors, totemic
connections, constitutive cosmologies, the presence of God, etc." (2010,
186). This is a "register of co-presence" that is representative of elements
that transcend constitutive sensoria. Indeed, in Liceti's investigation there
is an emphasis on the epi-phenomena of what goes on in Nature.

The engraving on folio 256r that features the "Papal Ass of Rome"
and the "monster of Krakow" is made all the more remarkable by the
presencing of additional, crudely drawn figures. One ill-defined figure
appears to be urinating on a monster with the head of a rabbit and a
severed umbilical cord hanging from the abdomen of a human-like body.
There also appears to be a winged griffin that is defecating while hanging
off the tail of the Krakow monster and being shot at by a winged figure.
A third griffin appears to be collecting the feces in a sack. Finally, the
monster with the rabbit head is being joined to the Krakow monster by
a spider weaving a web.

Beyond what is easily dismissed as nonsensical or disgusting about this engraving, it is important to understand that by the end of the sixteenth century, the "first stages of 'renaissance' grotesque style already has evolved into 'baroque'" (Barasch 1983, 60). The aesthetic of grotesquery was at the zenith of its popularity at the time Liceti was compiling *De Monstris* (Kayser 1966; Harpham 1976; Dorrian 2000). Furthermore, as Frances Connelly (2012) has shown, "the element of play" was the most pervasive feature of grotesque in this period. The term "grotesque" was used in reference to "fanciful works of extreme artifice and virtuosity" (Connelly 2012, 2). Furthermore, Connelly continues, the grotesque "is an action, not a thing—more like a verb than a noun. . . . Second, what the grotesque does best is to play or, rather, to put things into play. As visual forms, grotesques are images in flux: they can be aberrant, combinatory, and metamorphic" (2012, 2).

Together with the *tableau* of the three principal monsters a subnarrative of hunting monsters engaged in the acts of urination and defecation represents a *platea*. It is, I would argue, a visual space of interaction, guiding studious contemplation. It is a space that allows for an erasure of boundaries between a historical past and the reader's present. The grotesquery of urination and defecation are a counterpoint to the formal propriety of the grotesquery of the principal monsters. Following Mikhail Bakhtin, the reference to the bodily lower stratum of grotesquery may be seen to fulfill "a unifying, degrading, uncrowning and simultaneously regenerating function" (1984, 23). Further to this, I would like to add, it employs the operational principle of *lusus naturae* (i.e., a "joke of Nature").

> [A] discussion of *lusus* allows us to investigate aspects of pre-Linnaean taxonomy, in particular the need for alternative categories in classifying problematic phenomena, for *lusus* was frequently used as an anti-definition—a means of explaining something that would otherwise have been without explanation. . . . Jokes [of nature] are not self-evident; put in contemporary terms, they were an instance of the seemingly occult properties of nature made manifest through the discerning eye of the Renaissance naturalist. As such, *lusus* frequently distinguished more unusual phenomena from the quotidian. In other instances, it became an organizing principle that described the process of diversification in nature.
>
> (Findlen 1990, 293–294)

I am wholly in agreement here with Paula Findlen's assertion that "*lusus naturae*" should not be understood in the modern sense of a mischievous trick or a prank. It is not something said or done to evoke laughter or amusement. The phrase *lusus naturae* is generally translated in English to mean "a joke of Nature." But the word "*lusus*" literally means play or sports.

The analogical imagery used by natural philosophers in the seventeenth century reflects, in large part, the humanist "fascination with figurative language" (Findlen 1990, 294–295). Findlen indicates that following the Renaissance tradition of *serio ludere* (i.e., "to play seriously"), "the late Renaissance naturalists framed their reading of nature through a similar process of intellectual reversal and transformation that highlighted the paradoxes of the natural world" (Findlen 1990, 294).

Lusus "operated as a taxonomic principle, for it dissolved the difficulties of deciding in which category particularly subtle creations belonged by creating a space in which all of these irregular regularities could fit" (Findlen 1990, 303–304). This was a space flexible enough to accommodate all manner of what Francis Bacon had described as "deviating instances: such as the errors of nature, or strange and monstrous objects in which nature deviates and turns from her ordinary course" (quoted in Daston 2000, 16). More particularly, Connelly maintains that the organizational principle of grotesquery is revealed through its changes "in the interstitial moments when the familiar turns strange or shifts unexpectedly into something else" (2012, 3). If the grotesque has a structure, it is the structure of estrangement (Kayser 1966, 184). The grotesque is "in play"; it "always represents a state of change, breaking open what we know and merging it with the unknown" (Connelly 2012, 5). Furthermore, the naturalist as viewer is "pulled into a liminal space that both calls them into question and throws them open to possibility" (2012, 5–6).

The scenario and sub-narrative depicted in folio 236r lends insight into the way that *lusus naturae* operates as an organizing principle in Nature (see Figure 1.4). Here Lucas Cranach's Monk—Calf is placed next to a chimera with a "true bird's head" sitting on top of a human body. A sub-narrative of an angler landing a monster in the background calls attention to the event of "catching" a monster. The wonder of monstrousness is present *everywhere in Nature* and yet *we lose sight of it*. Instead, *we must catch sight of it* like an angler "catching" a monster. Once caught, we are in a better position to study and produce a taxonomy that can be linked to the kind of self-assured semiology that has been described as naturalized by early modern European science.

The space that is constructed for purposes of the anatomical dissection of monstrous births depicted in the Appendix of *De Monstris* is conspicuously vacuous (see Figure 1.5). All incidental details that might distract the reader from the concerns of practical *scientia* and *techne* have been blanked out and gotten rid of. A mechanical kind of objectivity is applied and what remains is what is intended to be *exempla* for scientific study and medical practice. This is a space in which the *serio ludere* of anatomy and learned medicine is organized. There is literally no backdrop to the birthing of children provided in the Appendix. The Appendix only offers a vision devoid of what Connelly has described as the

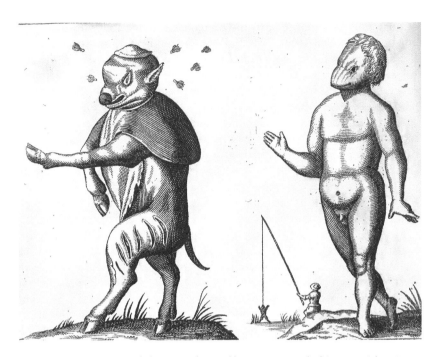

Figure 1.4 Engraving of the "Monk—Calf" monster and chimera with a "true bird's head" for Book II, folio 236r, *De Monstris* (1665). Amstelodami: Sumptibus Andreae Frisii, MDCLXV [1665]

Image courtesy of the Boston Medical Library.

"fundamental attributes of the grotesque (bodied, fertile, earth-bound, changeful) [which] align with those ascribed to the feminine" (2012, 2). In the end, the *lusus naturae* of giving birth is *mostly* left out of the picture. I say *mostly* because the Appendix includes one final engraving of conjoined twins on folio 316v which approaches the topic differently (see Figure 1.6). Here the twins appear to be performing, doing a balancing act on a cushion. The cushion marks, I would suggest, a boundary between the body of the twins and the site of their play. At the same time, the body of the twins is tied to their setting in terms of a relation of play that should not be mechanically detached from a perfectly natural event. *Lusus naturae*, Liceti seems to be reminding us, calls upon us to capture Nature's *ingenio* that both underpins and is the object of the *serio ludere* of medico-scientific investigation.

Conclusion: Reviewing Liceti's *De Monstris*

To sum up: I have argued that *lusus naturae* operates in *De Monstris* as an organizing principle to the extent that it both represents Nature's

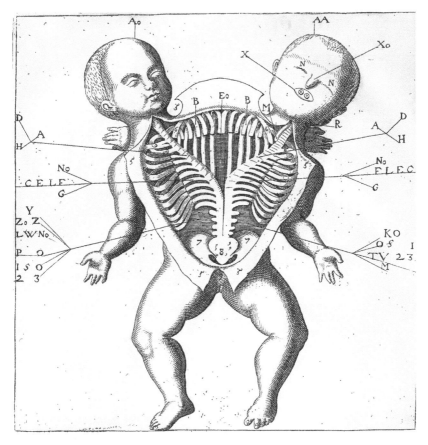

Figure 1.5 Engraving of conjoined twins for Appendix, folio 228r, *De Monstris*
(1665). Amstelodami: Sumptibus Andreae Frisii, MDCLXV [1665]

Image courtesy of the Boston Medical Library.

ingenio and supports the *serio ludere* of medico-scientific investigation.
I have said that the liminal space in which *lusus naturae* operates brings
with it the potential for breaking away from colloquial understandings
of empirical presence that typically exist in medico-scientific investigation. The assignment of normative judgments to particular monsters is
enacted within the boundaries of an order of knowing and doing. The
co-presence of *lusus naturae* and colloquial understandings of empirical
presence do not exist in *De Monstris* in a dichotomous relation to one
another. They are actually mutually constitutive of each other.

What is at stake, I submit, is a level of comprehension which is not easily
explained in a systematic way. *De Monstris* encourages us to apprehend

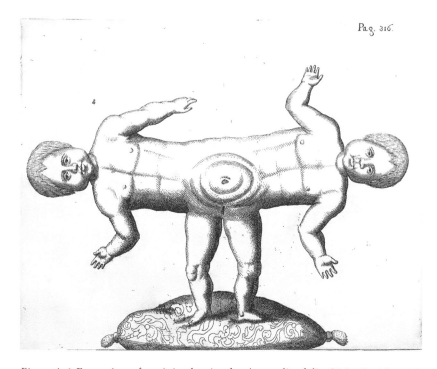

Pag. 316.

Figure 1.6 Engraving of conjoined twins for Appendix, folio 316v, *De Monstris* (1665). Amstelodami: Sumptibus Andreae Frisii, MDCLXV [1665]

Image courtesy of the Boston Medical Library.

the wondrous existence of monsters in Nature and it is the *ingenio* of Nature that is to be investigated through medico-scientific investigation. To do so, we must acknowledge a "register of co-presence" (*à la* Buchli) that must be attended to and this includes elements that transcend constitutive sensoria. Without doing so, we cannot fully appreciate the scope of *De Monstris* as an example of pre-Linnaean taxonomy linked to the self-assured semiology of naturalized early modern European science.

References

Ashworth, William B. 1990. "Natural History and the Emblematic World View." In *Reappraisals of the Scientific Revolution*, edited by David Lindberg and Robert Westman, 303–332. Cambridge: Cambridge University Press.

Bakhtin, Mikhail M. 1984. *Rabelais and His World*. Translated by H. Iswolsky. Bloomington: Indiana University Press.

Barasch, Frances K. 1983. "Definitions: Renaissance and Baroque, Grotesque Construction and Deconstruction." *Modern Language Studies* 13 (2): 60–67.

Bates, Alan W. 2001. "The De Monstrorum of Fortunio Liceti: A Landmark of Descriptive Teratology." *Journal of Medical Biography* 9: 49–54.

Bates, Alan W. 2005. *Emblematic Monsters: Unnatural Conceptions and Deformed Births in Early Modern Europe*. Amsterdam: Rodopi.

Blair, Ann. 2003. "Reading Strategies for Coping with Information Overload ca. 1550–1700." *Journal of the History of Ideas* 64 (1): 11–28.

Boylan, Michael. 1984. "The Galenic and Hippocratic Challenges to Aristotle's Conception Theory." *Journal of the History of Biology* 17: 83–112.

Bruner, Jerome. 1991. "The Narrative Construction of Reality." *Critical Inquiry* 18: 1–20.

Buchli, Victor. 2010. "Presencing the Im-Material." In *An Anthropology of Absence: Materializations of Transcendence and Loss*, edited by M. Bille, F. Hastrup, and T. Flohr Sørensen, 185–203. New York: Springer.

Canguilhem, Georges. 1962. "Monstrosity and the Monstrous." *Diogenes* 10 (40): 27–42.

Cheng, Sandra. 2012. "The Cult of the Monstrous: Caricature, Physiognomy, and Monsters in Early Modern Italy." *Preternature: Critical and Historical Studies on the Preternatural* 1: 197–231.

Connelly, Frances S. 2012. *The Grotesque in Western Art and Culture: The Image at Play*. Cambridge: Cambridge University Press.

Copenhaver, Brian P. 1990. "Natural Magic, Hermetism, and Occultism in Early Modern Science." In *Reappraisals of the Scientific Revolution*, edited by D. C. Lindberg and R. S. Westman, 261–302. Cambridge: Cambridge University Press.

Crowe, Norman. 1997. *Nature and the Idea of a Man-Made World: An Investigation into the Evolutionary Roots of Form and Order in the Built Environment*. Cambridge, MA: MIT Press.

Cusumano, Nicola. 2013. "'Fetal Monstrosities': A Comparison of Evidence from Sicily in the Modern Age." *Preternature: Critical and Historical Studies on the Preternatural* 2: 156–187.

Daston, Lorraine. 2000. "Preternatural Philosophy." In *Biographies of Scientific Objects*, edited by Lorraine Daston, 15–41. Chicago, IL: University of Chicago Press.

Daston, Lorraine, and Katharine Park. 1998. *Wonders and the Order of Nature*. New York: Zone.

Dorrian, Mark. 2000. "On the Monstrous and the Grotesque." *Word & Image* 16: 310–317.

Findlen, Paula. 1990. "Jokes of Nature and Jokes of Knowledge: The Playfulness of Scientific Discourse in Early Modern Europe." *Renaissance Quarterly* 43: 292–331.

Fisher, George Jackson. 1866. *Diploteratology: An Essay on Compound Human Monsters: Comprising the History, Literature, Classification, Description and Embryology of Double and Triple Formation, Including Parasitic Monsters, Foetus in Foetu, and Supernumerary Development*. Albany: Van Benthuysen's Steam Printing House.

Hampton, Timothy. 2004. "Signs of Monstrosity: The Rhetoric of Description and the Limits of Allegory in Rabelais and Montaigne." In *Monstrous Bodies/ Political Monstrosities: In Early Modern Europe*, edited by Laura Lunger Knoppers and Joan B. Landes, 179–199. Ithaca: Cornell University Press.

Harpham, Geoffrey. 1976. "The Grotesque: First Principles." *The Journal of Aesthetics and Art Criticism* 34: 461–468.

Henry, Devin. 2006. "Aristotle on the Mechanism of Inheritance." *Journal of the History of Biology* 39: 425–455.

Hsia, R. Po-chia. 2004. "A Time for Monsters: Monstrous Births, Propaganda, and the German Reformation." In *Monstrous Bodies/Political Monstrosities: In Early Modern Europe,* edited by Laura Lunger Knoppers and Joan B. Landes, 67–92. Ithaca: Cornell University Press.

Kayser, Wolfgang. 1966. *The Grotesque in Art and Literature.* New York: Columbia University Press.

Lazzarini, Elena. 2011. "Wonderful Creatures: Early Modern Perceptions of Deformed Bodies." *Oxford Art Journal* 34: 415–431.

Moscoso, Javier. 1998. "Monsters as Evidence: The Uses of the Abnormal Body during the Early Eighteenth Century." *Journal of the History of Biology* 31: 355–382.

Niccoli, Ottavia. 1990. *Prophecy and People in Renaissance Italy.* Translated by L. G. Cochrane. Princeton: Princeton University Press.

Ogilvie, Brian W. 2003. "The Many Books of Nature: Renaissance Naturalists and Information Overload." *Journal of the History of Ideas* 64: 29–40.

Ogilvie, Brian W. 2008. *The Science of Describing: Natural History in Renaissance Europe.* Chicago, IL: University of Chicago Press.

Randall, Michael. 1996. *Building Resemblance: Analogical Imagery in the Early French Renaissance.* Baltimore: Johns Hopkins University Press.

Stafford, Barbara Maria. 1999. *Visual Analogy: Consciousness as the Art of Connecting.* Cambridge, MA: MIT Press.

Verner, Lisa. 2016. *The Epistemology of the Monstrous in the Middle Ages.* London: Routledge.

Wittkower, Rudolf. 1942. "Marvels of the East: A Study in the History of Monsters." *Journal of the Warburg and Courtauld Institutes* 5: 159–197.

Wolfe, Charles T. 2005. "The Materialist Denial of Monsters." In *Monsters and Philosophy,* edited by C. T. Wolfe, 187–204. London: King's College Publications.

2   A Tlaxcalan Midwife's Toolkit

The Body, Medicine, Childbirth, and Contact Zone in Early to Mid-Colonial New Spain

Jacqueline Susann Holler

"Saint Anne gave birth a virgin, Saint Mary to Jesus Christ, Saint Elizabeth to Saint John. As these words are true I heal you from the evils of air, eye, art, and accident. Amen Jesus" (AGN 1652). In 1652, the *mestiza* (mixed-race) Tlaxcalan midwife and healer Isabel Hernández reported using these words to bless and cure her child patients—just one of many practice-based revelations contained in the record of her trial before the tribunal of the Holy Office in Mexico City. The incantation reported above might have arisen anywhere within the Catholic world, but other elements of Isabel's practice were clearly rooted in the soil of New Spain—and in understandings and *materia medica* drawn from the central Mexican indigenous medical tradition. In this chapter, I use Mexican Inquisition documents to gain partial but historically significant access to the world of colonial childbirth, a critical (and neglected) "contact zone." Mary Louise Pratt's (1991) seminal essay described colonialism in terms of the unprecedented and uncomfortable contact it produced between disparate groups of people. The contact zone, in Pratt's formulation, was the place where, in uneven and power-laden but often surprising exchanges, colonial cultures (and knowledge) were forged. Through examination of the case—and toolkit—of Isabel Hernández, I argue that childbirth was such a zone: an important locus for the transmission, forging, and transmutation of hybrid understandings of medicine and the body. My intent is not to deny the radical difference and, at times, mutual incomprehensibility of Iberian and Mesoamerican notions of embodiment, health, and medicine; nor do I wish to obscure the considerable divide between translation and meaning in cultural and linguistic exchange (Bassett 2015). That said, however, I argue that midwives and their clients bridged difference and shaped colonial understandings through the unavoidable work of birth—talking about, managing, and experiencing female bodies at the most liminal and fraught of moments. This chapter therefore offers a woman-, plebeian-, and body-centered corollary to recent studies that examine "heterogeneous knowledge" and areas of dialogue and crosspollination between European and indigenous learned traditions (*inter alia*, Diel 2016; Ramos and Yannakakis 2014).

Isabel Hernández was one of a relatively small number of midwives investigated for superstition and witchcraft between 1536 and the end of the eighteenth century. The resultant records have drawn some scholarly attention from historians of gender and witchcraft, such as Laura Lewis (2003) and Martha Few (2002), but have seldom been used as a source for the study of midwifery, medical practice, or childbirth itself. The few published studies of Mexican midwifery *per se* have been focused on regulation and the late colony and early republic. Luz María Hernández's (2018) recent volume on the nineteenth-century medical profession; John Tate Lanning's (1985) classic chapter on late colonial obstetrics; and Lee Penyak's (2002, 2003) work on the education and forensic activities of Mexican midwives in the late eighteenth and nineteenth centuries are important examples. Nora Jaffary's (2016) recent *Reproduction and Its Discontents* uses some Inquisition records, though its focus is the late colonial period and nineteenth century, and its emphasis the themes of birth control, abortion, and infanticide. Several works, however, have engaged with colonial feminine healing culture and medical tradition; Few's 2008 study applies the concept of "medical *mestizaje*" to Guatemala in the late colonial period, while Raquel Martín Sánchez (2005) has used a Colima Inquisition case to reconstruct the healing practices circulating in that city in the first half of the eighteenth century.

The paucity of midwifery studies, their emphasis on regulation, and their relatively late focus result from the attitude of colonial authorities toward the training and regulation of midwives. Provision for the licensing of midwives existed through the Royal Protomedicato, a regulatory body with deep Spanish (and indeed Roman) roots. However, just as the institution was formally extended to New Spain, it withdrew from responsibility for obstetrics; Philip II suspended its jurisdiction over midwives in 1567. Not until 1750 was there any effort to examine midwives (Lanning 1985; Hernández 2018). Only at the very end of the colonial period did interest in caesarean birth and obstetric reform illuminate the world of the Mexican midwife and begin the process that in other countries is referred to as the "medicalization" of birth.

Mexican midwifery's lack of a regulatory regime made it open to all comers and, thus, an exceptional example of colonial contact. On the other hand, the same absence of regulation and the concomitant lack of sources make the midwives of early colonial New Spain virtually impossible for the historian to identify. Hernández (2018, 89), for example, found only two licensed midwives for the whole colonial period, both in the eighteenth century. Lanning (1985) found that as late at 1830, there were only two licensed midwives in the entire Federal District of Mexico. Thereafter, licensing proceeded slowly: Jaffary (2016, 192) found a mere 24 midwives registered in Mexico City in 1866. Thus licensed midwives are virtually absent from the colonial (and early republican) archives of regulation. This makes it impossible to estimate the number of midwives in any given locality, let alone in the colony as a whole. Today, then, colonial Mexican childbirth, its personnel, and its role in bridging medical concepts and experiences of embodiment remain mysterious, particularly as regards the early colony. As an unintended consequence, virtually all studies of daily life, the family, women's lives, and death and dying in early colonial New Spain suffer from an absence of information related to childbirth: one of the most significant and frequent experiences of women, and one of the most significant spaces of contact among women (and some men) of diverse social location.

If regulatory documentation of colonial midwives is virtually nonexistent, Inquisition documentation is inconsistent but nonetheless suggestive. Of the roughly 2,400 Mexican Inquisition cases involving women, over 1,000 involve accusations of witchcraft and/or superstition, accusations almost certain to produce some information relative to healing (Martín Sánchez 2005). Through painstaking reading of these sources, I hope to reconstruct a picture of early colonial women's healing and embodiment. For this chapter, however, I have surveyed only cases from before 1660 in which women were identified as midwives. I refer only to cases in which the word "*partera*" was used; however, reliance on terminology such as this undoubtedly underrepresents the number of cases involving women who not only engaged in midwifery but were recognized as doing so by their communities (Martín Sánchez 2005). Nonetheless, the cases surveyed here demonstrate that the absence of regulatory oversight led many women to work and sometimes identify as midwives, increasing the number of women who practiced midwifery at least occasionally. For example, in April 1627, women in the small village of San Miguel de Culiacán (in northern New Spain) denounced five midwives, of whom four were currently practicing (AGN 1627a). Given the size of the community in question, one can surmise that there were many women who practiced midwifery on an irregular basis. Women's ability to move in and out of midwifery undoubtedly added to its heterogeneous nature.

Inquisition records also suggest that the unregulated, empirical nature of New Spain's midwifery increased its ethnic diversity. Many midwives, like Isabel Hernández, were women of mixed-race or African descent. It has sometimes been suggested that colonial ideas about non-Europeans as "closer to nature" may have increased the attractiveness of their healing services. For the early colonial period, however, arguably more important was the belief (rooted in Galenic medicine) that indigenous people were better able to understand and utilize the land and its *materia medica* (Earle 2012; Martínez Hernández 2014, 67–71). Whatever the case, though my sample of midwives is small, it is far from homogeneous. Of 11 early colonial midwives whose ethnic status I know, for example, three were "Spanish," five *mulata*, two *mestiza*, and one Black. "Spanish" women are thus quite well represented among the sample, while *mulata* women are overrepresented, characteristic of their wide representation in healing.

Though midwives identified as indigenous may appear largely absent from these Inquisition records, this absence reflects the Inquisition's lack of jurisdiction over indigenous people and cannot be assumed to indicate their absence from midwifery practice. Lisa Sousa (2017, 193–199) has examined the significance of Nahua female healers/midwives (*titiçih*) both before and during the colonial period. While female *titiçih* engaged in many forms of natural and supernatural healing (Pennock 2008, 41–47; Polanco 2018), they were recognized as birth experts in both indigenous and non-indigenous society. Thus midwifery was a truly *mestizo* realm in New Spain, with representation from all ethnic groups in the colony. Despite their plebeian status, midwives were also respected female professionals in both indigenous and Spanish settings—a far cry from their depiction as "ignorant *matronas*" by nineteenth-century medical men (Hernández 2018, 90). Some sense of midwives' status in colonial society can be gleaned from the fact that they are, with nuns and *beatas*, the only women identified by their trade (*oficio*) in Inquisition records. A professional group that commanded respect, deployed knowledge, and exhibited almost unique diversity, New Spain's midwives were well suited for the exchange and formulation of colonial medical knowledge.

Isabel Hernández first came to the Inquisition's attention after she was denounced, in Puebla, for "using, with evil and perverse intent, various powders, and committing other offences" (AGN 1652). Powders were ubiquitous in denunciations of superstition and witchcraft, and even now can be purchased in certain markets. The principal role of powders was to "tame," causing their consumer to be kindly disposed to, love, or obey the person who surreptitiously administered them. We should not be hasty to interpret Isabel's denunciation as evidence of distrust of midwives or conflation of the midwife with the witch. In contrast to the Guatemalan cases involving midwives examined by Few, Mexican cases do not generally appear to have arisen out of fears of malefice. Instead, *parteras* were usually denounced for specific practices identified as superstitious by particular edicts; witnesses make reference to having heard the edicts as motivation for coming forward, and cases make clear that superstitious practices were tolerated within the community until edicts catalyzed denunciation. A typical denunciation was that of Magdalena Cabeza de Vaca, a Spanish midwife resident in Mexico City, who was denounced because she apparently claimed the ability to accurately divine from an individual's palms "many things both present and future," in contravention of inquisitorial edicts (AGN 1626). While she had clearly engaged in her fortune-telling practice for some time without condemnation, the reading of an official edict produced denunciation in short order.

Seven witnesses testified against Isabel Hernández, six of them women between the ages of 20 and 60, and one a 50-year-old man. While noting Isabel's status as a midwife, the denunciations had nothing to do with childbirth and everything to do with the quotidian magic used by the women of New Spain. For example, the first witness to denounce Hernández, Inés de Herrera, described being in the *temazcal* (sweat lodge) with Hernández when a toad hopped out. Hernández urged Inés to take the toad and strangle it, promising to make a powder from the animal's body that would make any man "die for" Inés. Another woman described how her daughter had complained to Hernández at church about the stubbornness of the daughter's husband; Hernández, the witness claimed, had immediately offered the daughter (and later delivered) powders to "tame" the husband. Somewhat surprisingly, these denunciations were sufficient to result in a vote to arrest Hernández, sequester three trunks containing her belongings, and bring her to Mexico City for examination (AGN 1652).

Isabel Hernández did not know her age in 1652, but she appeared to the notary and inquisitors to be over 40. Born of a Castilian father and a *mestiza* mother descended from the indigenous nobility of Tlaxcala, Isabel was born in Guichiapa in the diocese of Tlaxcala in the central Mexican highlands. She was now resident in the city of Tlaxcala itself, where she housed with a local indigenous notable. This biography suggests a high degree of contact and mixing among Spanish, indigenous, and mestizo residents of the highlands. Indeed, Isabel's descriptions of her siblings suggest the degree of fluidity and "slipperiness" that Joanne Rappaport (2014) has found in the category "*mestizo*." Isabel's brother had married an indigenous woman, while Isabel's sister was married to a Spanish immigrant. Isabel herself had been married four times—each time to a Spanish immigrant—and had incorporated midwifery into a career that included not only her four marriages but a stint as a shopowner specializing in foodstuffs. Isabel was sufficiently well-regarded to have been called from the city to relatively remote parts approximately four times: she listed the clients she had visited in Guachinango (now Huauchinango, approximately 125 kilometers from Tlaxcala), three of whom bore the honorific "*doña*." She was also a mother of eight, with five children still living and several young grandchildren too. Isabel's family and social and professional networks thus comprised virtually the entire run of colonial society, from mixed-race plebeians to Spanish immigrants to Indigenous and Creole notables. Her medical practices and materials evince the same breadth.

Isabel's rootedness in indigenous healing practices was clear from the beginning of her case, when her friend Inés Herrera testified to conversations that occurred in the *temazcal*. The *temazcal*, or sweat lodge, was at the heart of central Mexican indigenous healing practices—as well as being a significant locus of colonial sociability.

Generally reckoned to be representative of the womb and primordial caves, the *temazcal* was under the protection of the mother of the gods (Bassett 2015). Colonial authorities sometimes associated the *temazcal* with diabolism and other illicit indigenous practices, but the sweat lodge was utilized throughout the colonial period for various forms of healing. The *temazcal* had a particularly important role in childbirth, as is indicated by the discussion in the *Florentine Codex:*

> Then one who has become pregnant, whose abdomen is already large, also enters there. There the midwives massage them; there they can place the babies straight in order that they will not extend crosswise nor settle face first. Two, three, four times they massage them there. And there those recently confined also bathe themselves; there, having delivered, having given birth, they strengthen their bodies. [The midwives] bathe them once, twice; and there they cleanse their breasts, that their milk will be good, and that they will produce a flow [of milk].
>
> (Sahagún 1963, 191)

The sweating induced by the lodge opened the body and created flow, the principal goal of indigenous medicine and one entirely compatible with the principles of Galenic medicine (as can be seen in the use of "humour" in the Spanish translation of Sahagún's Nahuatl text). Indeed, the core concept of Nahua healing—"that the body is a conduit and that one can take actions to keep it straight, clean, and in balance with the landscape and other people" (Stear 2015)—would have been almost entirely intelligible to non-indigenous Mexicans steeped in Galenism (Earle 2012; Duden 1991). In Central Mexican cosmovision and medicine, the human body acted as a pathway for divine energy, and the *temazcal* was a charged location for its transmission. Traditionally, birthing Nahua women commenced their labors in the *temazcal* and, in cases where there was no hope of delivery, were ceremonially enclosed there to die (Sousa 2017, 197). Because a neonate lacked its own *tonalli* (Polanco 2018) (often translated as "soul," but also comprehensible as "fire"), the warm *temazcal* was a healthy place to begin labor. After birth, the infant could be placed by a fire to await the moment when the *tonalli* entered the child's body (Furst 1995, 99–100). The *temazcal's* continued use by pregnant and birthing women and their newborns was documented in the early seventeenth century by the indigenous historian Chimalpahin. However, the persistence of the *temazcal* is often viewed as a *survival* of indigenous custom. The multiethnic *temazcal* culture glimpsed in Isabel Hernández's case suggests rather a diffusion and adaptation of indigenous healing in a broader, multiethnic colonial context.

Further revelations regarding Isabel's hybrid practice emerged through the course of her examination in Mexico City: in particular, when Isabel was eventually asked to detail the contents of her trunks and their uses. She described 17 items as they were presented to her. Some of Isabel's answers appear to the modern reader evasive, perhaps suggestive of dissembling; at the very least one would want to know more. For example, confronted with a small paw, appearing to be a monkey's, Isabel dismissed it as something her grandson had found in the square; a small stone idol was similarly dismissed. But whatever the limits of her explanations, Isabel's catalog gives a rare and uniquely comprehensive glimpse into the medical practice of a mid-colonial midwife—and into the considerable commingling and hybridization of Spanish and indigenous medical practices and conceptions of embodiment.

The first item in the catalog was an animal part. Describing the item as an opossum (*tlacuache*) tail, Isabel testified that she gave it to birthing women and to those with urinary problems: a use entirely consistent with pre-Columbian medical practice. The *Florentine Codex* notes the use of *tlacuache* tail as "a medicine which expels, which extracts, wherever something has gotten in"; "And [women] who have difficulty in childbirth, who cannot deliver the child, drink [the infusion]. Thus the little child is born quickly" (Sahagún 1963, 12). In addition to its vaunted expulsive properties, the tail of the opossum was reputed to ensure abundant lactation and to provoke sexual activity. One of the most venerated medicines in the Central Mexican indigenous tradition, *tlacuache* tail was known to non-indigenous Mexicans in the colonial period, indicating the mobility of knowledge and medicine across traditions (López Austin 1996, 301).

In addition to possessing a tail with acknowledged expulsive properties, the opossum was figured as intensely maternal. The opossum is not only a prolific mother but a competent and loving one: "Much does it squeal for its young. Much does it weep for them; true tears come forth. It places each in its pouch; it takes them out" (Sahagún 1963, 11–12). A marsupial (who therefore gives birth with ease), the *tlacuache* also appears to cheat death, since possums regularly "play dead" and then come back to life. At the risk of straining the evidence, one might assert that the *tlacuache*'s body had medico-magical power to cross the species barrier and infuse the birthing woman with the animal's own prolific and effortless motherhood.

Other indigenous components of Isabel's toolkit came from the central Mexican herbal tradition. The second item presented to her was described as a root, but she identified it as chichilpatle (*chichipatli*), identified by Sahagún as derived from tree bark and used as a purgative. Isabel said that she used it for infant indigestion or colic—again, a use consistent with the learned Nahua sources. A third item was identified as "some colored pieces" (AGN 1652). Isabel called them "*axi*" and described using them for women who are "stunned after childbirth." While their color might suggest that they were chiles (*ají*), it is also possible that they were actually axin, a fatty, lacquer-like substance made by the *coccus axinus* insect with similar uses in central Mexican medicine. Finally, Isabel was shown herbs that she identified as *cihuapatli* (or "woman herb"), which she said she administered to birthing women (AGN 1652).

Cihuapatli (*Montanoa tomentosa*), which stimulates powerful uterine contractions, was a potent medicine in the Central Mexican herbolary and of efficacy in both the second stage and, especially, the third stage of labor.

According to Sahagún:

> That which comes from its well-cooked foliage is required by the woman when she senses birth pains, when she is about to have a child. First the blood comes out, which shows that the baby is about to follow, about to be forced out. She is to drink it; wherewith she will quickly give birth. Thus she will not suffer much. It is to be drunk only once; but if the baby does not then follow, once again a little is to be drunk. Thus the baby can emerge.
>
> (1963, 180)

Not surprisingly, the herb was reputed to be (and is) a powerful abortifacient (Acosta et al. 1976, 84–86; Landgren et al. 1979); in the nineteenth century, medical men would become alarmed at the "abuse" of *cihuapatli* by Mexican women (Jaffary 2016, 84–86). This was of apparently little interest to the Inquisitors in Isabel Hernández' case, despite the fact that *cihuapatli* and its effects were already well known. Indeed, abortion appears in none of the early colonial cases examined for this chapter. This is surely not evidence of the absence of concern about abortion or the act itself. That concern, however, seems not to have attached itself to the midwives examined by the Holy Office in the early to mid-colonial period, perhaps because supplying such products fell to specialized traders. As both Laura Lewis (2003) and Serge Gruzinski (1993, 198–200) have shown, a thriving market for indigenous remedies and spells grew from the early colonial period on, integrating indigenous people into the market economy as purveyors of both natural and supernatural materials. It is no surprise, then, that in 1627 when 30-year-old *mestiza* Isabel de Ovando denounced herself for having attempted to procure an abortion for her daughter, she described asking an indigenous man, *not* a midwife, for a "potion to make the baby drop." In the event, Isabel lost her nerve when the practitioner told her that the house's holy images would have to be covered before the potion was administered (AGN 1627b). Clearly, early colonial plebeian women of all ethnicities were aware of the abortifacient possibilities contained in indigenous medical traditions—but midwives were not their first recourse when they sought such substances. By the late colonial period, this would change (Martín Sánchez 2005).

If numerous items in Isabel's toolkit appear transparently indigenous, her practice should not be interpreted as some form of nostalgic "cultural survival." First, even her use of indigenous medicines was hybridized. For example, she used the *tlacuache* tail by grinding it into powder and mixing it with warm pulque, fried onion, and almond oil—a decidedly colonial (and rather culinary) recipe, in contrast to the preparation of water, *tlacuache* tail, and chia described by Sahagún's informants (Sahagún 1963, 181). Moreover, Isabel's use of the *temazcal* was also influenced by the contact zone. There is no evidence, for example, that Isabel Hernández continued all aspects of the *temazcal* birthing tradition in her practice, such as the enclosure of a woman destined to die in childbirth. In fact, Isabel's case highlights the adoption of the *temazcal* outside the indigenous realm and its use by a *mestiza* midwife with a multiethnic clientele. Inés, the woman who initially denounced Isabel over the episode of the toad in the sweat lodge, was Spanish. Thus the *temazcal*, far from "surviving" among indigenous people, was at least tolerated by and arguably attractive to non-indigenous people, perhaps because of the complementarity between the indigenous concept of flow and the Galenic one.

Isabel's trial also demonstrates a concept of embodiment that appears to have moved in the opposite direction: from the Spanish world. After the midwife's arrest, a "principal Spanish maiden" (*donzella principal*) of the city reported a distressing situation that had occurred four years prior when Isabel was nursing the young woman's mother in her final illness. Upon the mother's death, Isabel had wrenched the teeth from the corpse's head. Confronted by a distressed servant and the woman's "stunned" daughters, Isabel told the women that she wanted the teeth "for relics," since she regarded the deceased woman as a saint (AGN 1652). It is well known that the European idea of the power of saintly body parts was highly influential in Mexico. Indeed, the cult of relics accorded well with preexisting indigenous concepts of bodily power, evident in human sacrifice and other central Mexican body rituals such as the *tlaquimolli* or sacred bundle, a frequent if elusive target of idolatry extirpations. During the colonial period, the *tlaquimolli* reincorporated and reanimated the god-body "so that she became, once again, an active agent living in the religious community" (Bassett 2015, 199). Perhaps influenced by this cross-fertilization of body traditions, Mexican "saints" had a habit of popping up like mushrooms after rain. The Mexican cult of relics had, perhaps, an even more "do-it-yourself" ethos than in contemporary Europe. For example, when the sixteenth-century missionary friar Motolinía died, his body had to be guarded closely because crowds attempted to tear relics from his corpse—a scene repeated in the early colonial period whenever saintly men and women died. Clearly Mexican relic culture, then, formed part of Isabel's practice. However, two facts are notable and suggestive: first, that witnesses described a careful wrapping of the teeth in paper at the time of their extraction, in terms faintly reminiscent of the *tlaquimolli*; and second, that the teeth were not found among Isabel's belongings by the Holy Office. A contact perspective cannot determine whether Isabel's extracted teeth inhered in indigenous, Catholic, or hybrid notions of bodily power but suggests the productive overlaps and dialogues that continued well into the colonial period.

Isabel's toolkit also contained other more clearly European items: small pieces of Venetian glass, used to make powders for women's faces, and "Ascension eggs," eggs gathered on the morning of the Feast of the Ascension 40 days after Easter. The Ascension eggs, along with the prayers and incantations used by Isabel according to her testimony, link the birthing woman's body to the bodies of Jesus Christ and his mother in a manner characteristic of late medieval and early modern European childbirth practice.

Isabel's apparent faith in relics and her use of the *temazcal* in healing reveal a fairly cohesive view of the body as both a conduit (in the Central Mexican tradition) and a vessel (in the Christian tradition) of sacred energy. That her practices and conceptions of the body were more syncretic than indigenous can also be seen in her toolkit, which included items of mystical or magical significance in the context of global science. For example, she possessed a *piedra bezoar*, or bezoar stone. The bezoar stone was discovered in Peru in the 1560s and became the subject of a sixteenth-century treatise (Stephenson 2010). Bezoars form inside the stomachs of ruminants, particularly South American camelids, and consist of undigested and calcinated coarse material that is eventually regurgitated or, frequently, removed from the animal after it is has been killed. When sufficiently large, such stones were known among the Inca as *ylla* (Holguín 1952 [1608], 366; Stephenson 2010). They were considered extremely valuable by both indigenous and non-indigenous people, so much so that one was presented to Philip II (Salomon 2004, 115). The term bezoar comes from the Persian word for anti-venom; it was believed that these magical American stones, which form inside mammalian bodies "like pearls in oysters," had capacity to neutralize poison (Bauer 2014, 81). While Isabel's bezoar was clearly unremarkable in size and her commentary upon it terse, the presence of the stone in her toolkit testifies to the circulation of medical materials within the Americas through colonial exchange. The evolving and heterogeneous medical marketplace clearly stretched not only between colonial capitals but into the Mexican highlands. There can be little doubt, therefore, of the hybridization not only of Iberian and Mesoamerican traditions, but of the incorporation of materials and practices from outside as well.

One final wondrous object in the toolkit was a little tusk on a cord, described by Isabel as a tooth of the "*pez mulier*" given to her by one of her sons. Reminiscent of the bezoar stone, the *pez mulier* was a marvelous New-World (Pacific) creature described as the "most rare fish, with a body half fish and half woman" (Leone 2016; Arita 2012; Bernabéu Albert 2006). Perhaps identifiable with the now-extinct Steller's sea cow, the *pez mulier* was an influential enough "discovery" to have stimulated its own medical industry. As a gift from son to mother, the tusk reinforced not only the power of the marvelous object but the connection and sympathy between woman and animal bodies. The use of animal parts (including marvelous or fictive ones) was well known in European medicine and even broader in the indigenous tradition, once again demonstrating the fusion between roughly complementary healing practices. Perhaps more importantly, Isabel's embrace of the bezoar and the *pez mulier* tusk demonstrates that New-World marvels, so often presumed to be a matter of metropolitan fascination, held allure for and were presumed powerful by mixed-race plebeians as well—and that colonial medicine had a cosmopolitan, even voracious appetite for healing novelties.

The emphasis of this chapter has been on Isabel Hernández's use of a heterogeneous toolkit. But what of her interlocutors, the inquisitors of Mexico City's Holy Office? As has already been mentioned, they showed remarkably little curiosity about any possible involvement in abortion, despite Isabel's possession of *cihuapatli*. Beyond this, however, Isabel's exposition of the contents of her trunk, examined, identified, and explained one at a time, appears to have been the decisive factor in her eventual release. Her escape from punishment (against the counsel of the clergymen who advised in the case) suggests that Isabel's medical knowledge counterbalanced more damning information about her sales of "powders." One cannot argue that the heterogeneous medical culture revealed in Isabel's testimony was therefore shared by the Inquisitors of the Holy Office, but at the very least their actions in the case suggest a modicum of respect.

While the study of one plebeian midwife's toolkit cannot reveal the entirety of birthing practice in the early colony, the chests owned by Isabel Hernández reveal much about the ways in which early colonial midwives healed. Isabel's toolkit demonstrates that a multiethnic birthing and medicinal tradition was accessible to and used by colonial midwives; moreover, her case reveals how this tradition is evident in Inquisition documents even when those documents are not primarily concerned with midwifery-related issues. In sum, then, colonial Mexican midwifery was a hybrid realm, both Spanish and *casta*, drawing from multiple medical and herbal traditions, blurring the ever-porous boundaries between medicine and magic, and confounding historical binaries. As a realm of exploration, empiricism, and intimate contact among diverse colonial subjects, it produced new forms of colonial embodiment whose traces remain in popular Mexican medicine today. The investigation of medical hybridization in the lives of plebeians is a fruitful avenue for exploring the broader cultural processes that confound the knowledge categories of colonial society.

References

Acosta, Mariclaire, Flora Botton Burlá, Lilia Domínguez, Isabel Molina, Adriana Novelo, and Kyra Núñez. 1976. *El aborto en México*. Mexico: Fondo de Cultura Económica.

AGN (Archivo General de la Nación, Mexico). 1626. Ramo Inquisición, Vol. 360, 1a parte, f. 7. Mariana de la Cruz contra Magdalena Cabeza de Vaca. Translated by the author.

AGN. 1627a. Ramo Inquisición, Vol. 360, 2a parte. Denunciación que hizo de sí Catalina González, f. 483; Denunciación de Costanza Maldonado que hizo de sí, f. 488; Denunciación de Inés de Xerez contra Catalina González, partera, f. 488v; Denunciación de Doña María de Maldonado contra unas parteras, f. 484.

AGN. 1627b. Ramo Inquisición, Vol. 360, 1a parte, f. 469. Isabel de Ovando contra sí.

AGN. 1652. Ramo Inquisición, Vol. 561, 1a y 2a partes. Exp. 6, ff. 525–568. Proceso causa crim^l contra Isabel Hernandez biuda n^l de Gueichiapa de oficio partera i curandera, vez^a de Tlax^a obpado de la Puebla. Translated by the author.

Arita, Hector. 2012. "El Pez Mulier." *Mitología Natural*. Last modified February 16. https://hectorarita.com/2012/02/16/el-pez-mulier/

Bassett, Molly H. 2015. *The Fate of Earthly Things: Aztec Gods and God-Bodies*. Austin: University of Texas Press.

Bauer, Ralph. 2014. "The Blood of the Dragon: Alchemy and Natural History in Nicolás Monardes's *Historia Medicinal*." In *Medical Cultures of the Early Modern Spanish Empire*, edited by John Slater, Maríaluz López-Terrada, and José Pardo-Tomás, 67–90. Farnham, UK/Burlington, VT: Ashgate.

Bernabéu Albert, Salvador. 2006. "Una mirada científica a la frontera: California en la centuria ilustrada." *BROCAR* 30: 15–36.

Diel, Lori Boornazian. 2016. "The *Codex Mexicanus*: Time, Religion, History, and Health in Sixteenth-Century New Spain." *The Americas* 73 (4): 427–458.

Duden, Barbara. 1991. *The Woman Beneath the Skin: A Doctor's Patients in Eighteenth-Century Germany*. Translated by Thomas Dunlap. Cambridge, MA/London: Harvard University Press.

Earle, Rebecca. 2012. *The Body of the Conquistador: Food, Race, and the Colonial Experience in Spanish America, 1492–1700*. Cambridge: Cambridge University Press.

Few, Martha. 2002. *Women Who Live Evil Lives: Gender, Religion, and the Politics of Power in Colonial Guatemala*. Austin: University of Texas Press.

Furst, Jill Leslie McKeever. 1995. *The Natural History of the Soul in Ancient Mexico*. New Haven/London: Yale University Press.

Gruzinski, Serge. 1993. *The Conquest of Mexico: The Incorporation of Indian Societies into the Western World, 16th–18th Centuries*. Translated by Eileen Corrigan. Cambridge, MA: Polity Press.

Hernández, Luz María. 2018. *Carving a Niche: The Medical Profession in Mexico, 1800–1870*. Montreal: McGill-Queen's University Press.

Holguín [González Holguín], Diego. 1952 [1608]. *Vocabulario de la lengua general de todo el Peru llamada lengua Qquicha o del Inca*, edited by Raúl Porras. Lima: Instituto de Historia, Universidad Nacional Mayor de San Marcos.

Jaffary, Nora. 2016. *Reproduction and Its Discontents in Mexico: Childbirth and Contraception from 1750 to 1905*. Chapel Hill: University of North Carolina Press.

Landgren, Britth Marie, Kerstin Hagenfeldt, and Egon Diczfalusy. 1979. "Clinical Effects of Orally Administered Extracts of *Montanoa Tomentosa* in Early Human Pregnancy." *American Journal of Obstetrics and Gynecology* 135 (4): 480–484.

Lanning, John Tate. 1985. "Government and Obstetrics." In *The Royal Protomedicato: The Regulation of the Medical Profession in the Spanish Empire*, edited by John Jay TePaske, 298–324. Durham: Duke University Press.

Leone, Massimo. 2016. "Travel, Monsters, and Taxidermy: The Semiotic Patterns of Guillibility." *Religación: Grupo de Investigaciones en Ciencias Sociales y Humanidades desde América Latina* 1 (1): 9–26.

Lewis, Laura. 2003. *Hall of Mirrors: Power, Witchcraft, and Caste in Colonial Mexico*. Durham: Duke University Press.

López Austin, Alfredo. 1996. *Los mitos del tlacuache: Caminos de la mitología mesoamericana*. Mexico: UNAM.

Martínez Hernández, Gerardo. 2014. *La medicina en la Nueva España, siglos XVI y XVII*. Mexico: UNAM.

Martín Sánchez, Raquel. 2005. *Hechiceras en la Colima novohispana*. Colima: Universidad de Colima, Cuadernos ACU.

Pennock, Caroline Dodds. 2008. *Bonds of Blood: Gender, Lifecycle and Sacrifice in Aztec Culture*. Basingstoke, UK/New York: Palgrave MacMillan.

Penyak, Lee. 2002. "Midwives and Legal Medicine in Mexico, 1740–1846." *Journal of Hispanic Higher Education* 1 (3): 251–266.

Penyak, Lee. 2003. "Obstetrics and the Emergence of Women in Mexico's Medical Establishment." *The Americas: A Quarterly Review of Inter-American Cultural History* 60 (1): 59–85.

Polanco, Edward Anthony. 2018. "'I Am Just a Tiçitl': Decolonizing Central Mexican Nahua Female Healers, 1535–1635." *Ethnohistory* 65 (3): 441–463.

Pratt, Mary Louise. 1991. "Arts of the Contact Zone." *Profession*: 33–40.

Ramos, Gabriela, and Yanna Yannakakis, eds. 2014. *Indigenous Intellectuals: Knowledge, Power, and Colonial Culture in Mexico and the Andes*. Durham: Duke University Press.

Rappaport, Joanne. 2014. *The Disappearing Mestizo: Configuring Difference in the Colonial New Kingdom of Granada*. Durham: Duke University Press.

Sahagún, Bernardino de. 1963. *General History of the Things of New Spain (Florentine Codex), Book 11-Earthly Things*. Translated by Charles E. Dibble and Arthur Andersen. Salt Lake City: University of Utah Press.

Salomon, Frank. 2004. "Andean Opulence: Indigenous Ideas about Wealth in Colonial Peru." In *The Colonial Andes: Tapestries and Silverwork 1530–1830*, edited by Elena Phipps, Johanna Hecht, and Cristina Esteras Martín, 114–124. New York: Metropolitan Museum of Art.

Sousa, Lisa. 2017. *The Woman Who Turned into a Jaguar and Other Narratives of Native Women in Archives of Colonial Mexico*. Stanford: Stanford University Press.

Stear, Ezekiel. 2015. "Beyond the Fifth Sun: Nahua Teleologies in the Sixteenth and Seventeenth Centuries." Ph.D diss., University of Kansas. www.academia.edu/34941184/BEYOND_THE_FIFTH_SUN_NAHUA_TELEOLOGIES_IN_THE_SIXTEENTH_AND_SEVENTEENTH_CENTURIES

Stephenson, Marcia. 2010. "From Marvelous Antidote to the Poison of Idolatry: The Transatlantic Role of Andean Bezoar Stones during the Late Sixteenth and Early Seventeenth Centuries." *Hispanic American Historical Review* 90 (1): 3–39.

3 Ecstasies, Stigmata, and Visions

Body and Sanctity in *La Civiltà Cattolica* in the Age of Positivism (1888–1890)

Carlo Bovolo

In the course of the nineteenth century and particularly in its second half, science began to have a growing influence on Italian society and culture. At the same time, it threatened the authority and the influence of the Church and of Catholicism in Italy, which were in turn already under pressure because of the slow but gradual secularization and the national unification process under the Kingdom of Sardinia's Liberal-Monarchic guide (1861), leading to the end of the pope's temporal power with the conquest of Rome (1870). The centrality of science in the nineteenth century, moreover, put Catholics up against the question of how to react to and face modernity, whose strength lay in science and in the positive method, in order to safeguard the role of the Church and Catholic orthodoxy. Hence the spreading in some sectors of the Catholic movement, especially in some clerical periodicals, of the need to build a science in accordance with Revelation, with the idea of developing strategies to embrace scientific matters through a Christian perspective, to respond to the lay and positivist materialistic theories of scientists, to strengthen the Catholic public opinion also in the sciences, and to strive for a scientific dissemination harmonized with faith.

Science and medicine became significant and effective instruments at the service of the Catholic propaganda, used by the clerical press with impetus. The importance given to the medicine and the efforts to develop an apologetic narrative and to organize the public presence of Catholic physicians and scientists stemmed not only from the increasing importance of the biological and physiological data in cultural policies, social welfare, and health of the nineteenth century, but also from the belief that science could be used effectively in one of the major controversies that opposed Catholics and positivists in the second half of the century: the debates on the origin and authenticity of miracles, wonders, relics, and divine signs (such as apparitions, ecstasies, stigmata, and healings).

The attention toward phenomena not immediately and easily understandable and explainable in relation to man and to the human body was a constant in nineteenth-century science, involving both Catholics and the positivist and materialist laity. It is in the nineteenth century that the first scientific studies of the human psyche and its pathologies were conducted (from Jean-Martin Charcot's research on hysteria to Cesare Lombroso's studies on deviance and crime), while there also spread a series of pseudo-scientific phenomena and practices (such as mesmerism, magnetism, hypnotism, and spiritualism) that sparked fierce debates.

In the course of the nineteenth century, practices of animal magnetism, hypnotism, and somnambulism, generated by the common theme of mesmerism at the end of the eighteenth century,[1] were remarkably diffuse, proving to be successful and hence attracting the whole of Europe's interest, so much so that it became a true cultural fashion. The phenomena related to the currents of magnetism and hypnotism were the subject of lively debates, in a position constantly balanced between science, imposture, and the supernatural. Magnetism represented a sort of third way, as opposed to religion and science, presenting itself as alternative and antagonistic to both (Armando 2013). The Church had to inevitably face the magnetic and hypnotic phenomena. In 1840, the Holy Office expressed a negative opinion, albeit without publicizing openly this condemnation of magnetism, for reasons of caution and in order not to further advertise the practices, then reconfirmed the judgment of illicitness on further occasions (1841, 1843, 1847). In 1856, the Pope Pius IX denounced the abuses of magnetism, an offshoot of superstition, and in the 1860s the works of the hypnotist and spiritualist Allan Kardec were listed in the *Index librorum prohibitorum*. Whilst the Church's official approach was somewhat cautious, there was a stronger opposition by the Catholic press that throughout the second half of the century brought forward a heated dispute. Although they acknowledged the existence of charlatans and quacks, the Catholic apologists, who had more freedom of action compared to the ecclesiastical institutions, did not even deny the possibility of supernatural phenomena, as did the skeptics, nor did they welcome with curiosity and interest the phenomena that they could not control, as did some eminent scientists, such as the criminal anthropologist Cesare Lombroso and the psychiatrist Enrico Morselli. Catholics strongly argued with these positivistic scientists who stubbornly and vainly sought, in nature and in matter, a rational explanation. In recognizing the existence of supernatural phenomena, but not being able to reconnect them with the supernatural of divine origin (such as miracles, apparitions, etc.), the Catholic point of view was calling into question demonology-related explanations, harshly criticizing these practices, because of their evil nature and their opposition to Catholic principles (e.g., doubting free will).

In this cultural climate, where positivist science aimed to debunk deception and to rationally explain phenomena that were interpreted as supernatural, Catholics felt the need for a counteroffensive. It involved the defense of manifestations of alleged divine origin, from Marian apparitions to prodigious relics, from miraculous healings to the stigmata that renewed the martyrdom of Christ on the bodies of presumed saints. The development of a Catholic scientific discourse in the second half of the nineteenth century offered new apologetic opportunities, which allowed questioning the authenticity and highlighting the limitations of rationalist science and its inadequacy, thus demonstrating the indispensable role of faith even in scientific and medical matters.

A series of articles that appeared in *La Civiltà Cattolica* between July 1888 and May 1890, represented for Italian Catholics a fundamental point of reference in the complex relationship between the supernatural and science, and between holiness and medicine concerning the body. Founded in 1850, *La Civiltà Cattolica*, the Italian Jesuit periodical, was a faithful reflection of the Church's positions, and a laboratory and reference point of intransigent Catholic thought, with the aim of defending the role of the Pope and the principles of Catholicism, hence putting in place a program of apologetic and propaganda commitments (Traniello 2007; Forno 2012). The articles contained a thorough analysis of phenomena and bodily signs considered to be of divine origin—but put in doubt by positivists—that science would have been able to explain, if it was guided by faith. The author was the Jesuit Francesco Salis Seewis, in charge, for the last quarter of the century, of scientific matters in the editorial staff of *La Civiltà Cattolica*. The articles were published again in 1892 in an extended version in two volumes: *Le estasi, le stigmate e la scienza* and *Visioni e allucinazioni*.

In the middle of the century, several apparition episodes, particularly Marian ones, and phenomena of presumed supernatural origin, such as stigmata and divine ecstasies (Belgian Louise Lateau's being the most notorious case), sparked lively debates both within the Catholic world and in the scientific community. During the nineteenth century, moreover, Marian devotion had a considerable impetus, strengthened by the proclamation of the dogma of the Immaculate Conception on 8 December 1854. For this reason, the episodes of the apparitions of Virgin Mary had a wide resonance at an international level, particularly with the best known cases of La Salette in Isère (in 1846; the apparitions were recognized by the Church in 1851), of Lourdes (in 1858; recognized by the local bishop already in 1862), and Marpingen in Germany (in 1876; never recognized and then discovered to be an act of deception).

Apparitions and visions, miraculous healings, Christly wounds on the body of presumed saints, episodes of hypnotism and Donatism, research on hysteria and on psychiatric disorders and neurological diseases in general, the application of the positive method for the investigation: all these factors drove the Jesuit periodical to become involved in a complex and thorny issue, implementing its doctrinal authority and its apologetic power. Although dedicated to ecstasies, visions, and stigmata, as divine signs and possible clues of holiness, the series of articles intended to give an orthodox and quasi-official interpretation both of past episodes on which the Church had not expressed an opinion and, above all, of future cases.

The magazine started by making a conceptual distinction between the attention gained by the latest discoveries and by the most recent medical findings and the one addressing hysteria: in the first case it was to disclose the origins and treatments of the pathologies; in the second case,

> all the noise, instead, brought about by the hysterology observations, proceeds from the pride that the incredulous demonstrate in having found in this morbid disease a natural explanation of the phenomena already assigned to either diabolical obsession or to supernatural graces, such as ecstasies, visions, revelations, stigmata, and many miracles. Hence the representation of the Church as convinced, by scientific progress, of a shameful blunder in both the institution of its exorcisms, and in the acknowledgement of those so-called graces conceded for free; not only the Church, but Scripture itself, in the story of visions and revelations, and presumed freeing of the obsessed, operated by Jesus Christ and his disciples.
>
> (Salis Seewis 1888, 267–268)

The argumentative cue of the article was provided by the definition of *exstase*, compiled by the French doctor and alienist Claude-François Michéa (1815–1882), in the *Dictionnaire de médecine et de chirurgie*: according to the current positivistic medical interpretation, ecstasy was considered a state of disease, the origins of which were "strong commotions, fears, upset love, scientific and literary enthusiasm, and especially religious sentiment" (Salis Seewis 1888, 269), but without the intervention of any supernatural element, however implicitly referring to superstition and fanaticism. Citing several cases in which ecstatic episodes were evaluated by physicians as a result of hysteria or other nervous disorders, the magazine observed that "modern medicine shows, in this field, a little too hasty and, at the same time, a more pedantic diagnosis than is deserved in a topic that is not wholly within its domain" (1888, 273). *La Civiltà Cattolica* did not doubt the existence of these nerve diseases, but noted that:

> The modern conclusions, in so far as they relate to the existence of morbid ecstasies, repeat a fact that is well known by medicine of the past centuries, and was always taken into consideration by theologians and the Church; which, however, does not lessen at all the deference, whence theologians themselves welcome new medical observations, at the mercy of which the causes of nervous ecstasies are more clearly determined. But when modern medicine, or whoever takes on its interpretation, ventures to state that never in history are ecstasies or visions either shown or have been shown

to be of any nature other than hysterical and without a shadow of supernatural intervention, it is obvious that Aesculapius's followers are passing from a positive analysis of the facts to a general and exclusive assertion: in such a passage, induction teaches us to doubt whether the qualification as doctors may prevent them sufficiently from making any serious blunder.

(1888, 273)

As long as medicine concerned itself with episodes of nervous diseases, the Church, in its attentive mission to mind the health of the faithful, had no issues. But when physicians, such as Henri Legrand de la Saulle, a colleague of Charcot's in Paris, stated that many blessed women and saints were nothing more than hysterical, the situation changed, and it was therefore necessary to intervene. To demonstrate that the cases of religious ecstasies could not be explained pathologically, the article described hysteria in detail, thence proceeding to a comparison between the characteristics that medicine recognized as belonging to nervous disease and religious ecstasies. The Jesuits, in other words, used the same scientific arguments to rule out a pathological cause and consequently reinforce the rather particular and therefore divine origin of mystical ecstasies.

First of all, the age of the patients was considered: according to physicians, hysterical crises ended at 40 or 50 years of age, so they were deemed a disorder typical of adolescence and youth. The article thus pontificated: "In a word: [positivist scientists had] to either retract the influence of advanced age on hysteria or to confess that in a good diagnosis the ecstasies in Christian hagiography cannot be explained as being a whole with the hysteria hypothesis" (Salis Seewis 1888, 34). But since there was a broad consensus among doctors on this point, there was no other choice but to observe that "the assumption of hysteria in Christian hagiography ecstasies was contradicted by medicine itself" (1888, 35). Secondly, the rarity of documented cases of hysteria in the unmarried, particularly among the religious, was invoked. Finally, since it was envisaged that hysteria originated from an irregular lifestyle, "not accustomed to restraining passions," from this point of view "the Saints of Christian martyrology provide the physician with the most opposite diathesis for the presumption of hysteria" (1888, 35). Almost as if anticipating an objection, *La Civiltà Cattolica* prepared itself by pointing out that the Church did not systematically canonize all those who had episodes of ecstasies; on the contrary, medicine played a fundamental role in observing the phenomena's pathological or natural origin thanks to a careful medical analysis of the body and the morals:

> The Church, before raising a Servant of God to the altars, thus authenticating, indirectly and generally, the ecstasies, if ever she had any,

ensures an extremely accurate process to assess that there were no symptoms that may be ascribed by modern medicine to a hysterical inclination. It is quite clear that there cannot be the pretense from us that the Church in its process of beatification put the question in these terms: whether, in other words, the Servant of God showed symptoms of hysteria; but just as clear is the fact that the Church wants a demonstration in those processes, firstly, that the ecstatic occurrence be free from those depraved inclinations, that inextricably accompany hysteria; and not only that it be free, but that it showed opposing inclinations of an extraordinary degree and, using a most appropriate expression, of a heroic degree.

(1888, 35–36)

Based on this, the belief that the ecstasies narrated by Christian hagiography were simple cases of hysteria, was a judgment "intertwined with contradictions and inconsistencies" (1888, 50). And, further on, it was reiterated: "if there ever was a hypothesis badly crafted by rationalists against supernatural phenomena, it is this one, seeking to reduce Christian ecstasies to hysterical affections. It doesn't hold together either for the Saintly women for whom it was badly fit, or for the Saints on whom it fits just like a female garment on a man" (Salis Seewis 1888, 413).

Salis Seewis explicitly argued against *Le estasi umane* recently published by Paolo Mantegazza (1831–1910), a positivist and materialist, evolutionist, and anticlerical founder of anthropology in Italy. Written after the controversy raised by *Gli amori degli uomini* (1871), "a work for a brothel" that fell "in the murky and foul quagmire of human vices" (Salis Seewis 1889–1890, 8), in *Le estasi umane*, the anthropologist, gathering some of the reflections made during a journey in Scandinavia, proposed now to "climb to the highest summits of thought and sentiment, where man arrives heaving and breathless, but blessed to have climbed so high" (Mantegazza 1887, 3–5). The work, according to the review of the Jesuit, "while mentioning the rise to the highest summits of thought and sentiment, at every step stumbles, with a lewd and lubricious telling, drenching its pages in its beloved quagmire" while its author "dogmatizes as a non-believer and defines as a materialist" (Salis Seewis 1889–1890, 9–10). Mantegazza's book actually only mentioned the medical field briefly, referring mainly to the objects of ecstasies, understood as a strong attenuation of thought or an exaltation of affection: friendship, maternal love, contemplation of nature, but also patriotic love. As was explained by the title itself and in accord with his beliefs, the anthropologist author denied any supernatural elements, reducing them to mere human phenomena. Therefore, in the gallery of ecstatic figures, there appeared, side by side, St. Teresa of Avila and the Count of Cavour, a mother and a Platonic lover. Mantegazza's intent was, indeed, to emphasize the common human nature of different types of ecstasies. However, the article specifically highlighted how a juxtaposition between the ecstatic Teresa of Avila and the other figures showed, contrary to what the anthropologist claimed, the origin and the special nature of the ecstasy of the former, "a woman, who flying over the world of the senses, fades into the invisible sun of Divinity: and where the most solid minds beg for the concepts and timidly weigh the terms, she, a woman without any further education than a devout young nun, proceeds with sureness, like someone reading an invisible book without ever encountering improprieties or errors" (Salis Seewis 1889–1890, 11–12). Highlighting the limits of science and claiming "the absolute difference that runs between the two psychological phenomena, bundled here under the name of ecstasies," Salis Seewis stated that the human ecstasies, cited by Mantegazza, could not be defined and that only "the ecstasy of Saint Teresa and other Saints is ecstasy, but it is not human in every part: here there is, no doubt, something of the supernatural" (Salis Seewis 1889–1890, 13). Regarding an interpretation of the phenomenon as seen through hypnotism, proposed among others even by Mantegazza, the article kept its distance, once again reiterating the divine nature of true ecstasies in addition to highlighting the differences:

> What has this got to do with the sequel of ever deeper dreams with the increasing activity of an ecstatic soul, that with all the ardour of its many cognitive powers enters into the sight and love of the heavenly things? And those states of sleep reduced to a method, prepared by an appropriate education, depending on a command from an operator, and that approach proper sleepwalking; what do they have to do with the ecstatic raptures, often of sudden nature, not even preceded by an inner collection, and determined only by a mysterious force that raises the soul and raptures it to exercise the highest of its powers? . . . All together the hypnotizers of the world will never produce an ecstatic, for the simple reason that sleepwalking is a diametrically opposite state compared to that of ecstasy.
>
> (Salis Seewis 1889–1890, 17)

The hypnotic phenomena, which were the result of charlatanism or, worse still, of demonic nature, had nothing to do with the mystical ecstasies of divine nature, so much so that "true ecstasy is not a human thing, and we adjust for completion the inverse proposition, that human ecstasies are a chimera" (Salis Seewis 1889–1890, 24).

After having distinguished the only real form of ecstasy, the mystical one of divine origin, from other forms, Salis Seewis addressed another topic that had sparked the debates both in the scientific and Catholic worlds: the episodes of stigmata appearances. The topic centered the debate on the relationship between body and holiness: the wounds that marked the body recalling the wounds received by Christ represented an indisputable mark of holiness; and medicine itself, called into question, could sanction its divine origin, as it failed to identify a natural and pathological cause. The obvious reference for the public, at the end of the nineteenth century, was the famous case of Louise Lateau (1850–1883). The sequence of events of the young Belgian, who in addition to being affected by mystical ecstasies, displayed the Christly wounds from 1868 to 1881, became famous throughout Europe, and sparked a lively debate in the press and in scientific institutions, as recently illustrated by Gabor Klaniczay (2013). To assess the case, in 1868, the bishop of Tournai and the Archbishop of Malines, Victor-Auguste Dechamps, had already appointed a medical and ecclesiastic committee, formed, among others, by Ferdinand Lefebvre, a physician from Louvain and promoter of a Catholic scientific society in 1875, and by Antoine Imbert-Gourbeyre, a doctor and fervent Catholic, known to Catholic readers for his interventions on pastoral hygiene and medicine. The commission, presided by Lefebvre, concluded after a year of observations that medical science was not able to scientifically explain the stigmata, the origin of which should therefore be supernatural (Lefebvre 1870). A cult very quickly developed around Louise Lateau's persona and her body, at first locally, and then even internationally, acknowledging the young girl to be a saint. Many books, pamphlets, and printed pictures were published and spread across Europe. The climate of Catholic and Marian devotion revival and, at the same time, the electoral confirmation of the Catholic party in Belgium in 1870, which took advantage of devotional traditions and cults for its political and cultural rooting, contributed to Lateau's cult. The case was once again brought to the attention of the community of scientists and the public by the investigations and by the debates that engaged physicians and scientists at the Académie royale de médecine de Belgique, resulting in an international resonance. In July 1874, Nestor Charbonnier, a member of the academy, linked the stigmata to anorexia and insomnia (Lateau stated she had not eaten or slept since 1871), indicating the cause of the permanent wounds in the physiological food and sleep deprivation (Charbonnier 1875). In September, Rudolf Virchow (1874), a scientific authority in the pathological and physiological fields, at a conference in Wrocław, expressed his skepticism about the case, also because of the family's and clergy's firm opposition to an observation of the young girl in a laboratory. A similar opinion was expressed in October by Hubert Boëns (1875), a Charleroi doctor specializing in hygiene and public health. The Belgian Academy decided to appoint Évariste Warlomont to proceed with a new investigation: in confirming the spontaneous nature of the wounds, Warlomont (1875), however, assigned the cause to the action of the imagination on the nervous system, rejecting any supernatural explanation. The debate continued in the Belgian press with accusations addressed to Catholic superstition and to Lefebvre, in turn defended by the Catholic newspapers, and with a new scientific interpretation of the phenomenon proposed by a pupil of Charcot's, Désiré Bourneville Magloire (1875), which was centered on hysteria and openly anticlerical.

The case of the stigmatized girl from Bois d'Haine had an international resonance, even in Italy: in 1872, Father Antonio Pellicani (1872), a teacher at the Collegio degli Artigianelli of Turin, wrote a biography of Louise Lateau that retraced Henri Van Looy's life, while, in 1879, the Piedmontese priest Lorenzo Trecco (1879) included the episode in the second volume of *Avvenimenti meravigliosi antichi e recenti*, together with the Marian apparitions of La Salette and Lourdes. Regarding the press, the echoes of the controversy about the authenticity of Lateau's stigmata appeared in *L'Unità Cattolica*, the intransigent Catholic newspaper that was most attentive to the anticlerical controversies coming from north of the Alps. Defending the divine miracle, the newspaper attacked materialist science and the incredulity of its followers:

> All the weakness of superb modern science in front of religion is manifested in the discussions that take place amongst the doctors in Belgium on Louise Lateau's stigmata in Bois d'Haine. Mr. Warlomont and several colleagues who profess materialism, having been able to convince themselves, with a scrupulous examination of the facts, that there was no abuse whatsoever, and not wanting to confess a miracle, have concluded it must be a 'stigmatic neuropathy' . . . so the incredulous, who find a miracle absurd, must instead believe to be natural fact that now, for seven years, every Friday, at the same time, the hands and the feet and the rib cage of Louise Lateau receive the stigmata of the Divine Savior's wounds! Thirty years ago, there were scientists who were certain in their denial of the stigmata of Saint Francis; now they cannot deny the similar fact, and therefore come up with 'stigmatic neuropathy.' The day will come in which they will recognize their ignorance.
>
> ("I materialisti e le stimmate" 1875)

The notoriety of the Lateau case had put forward questions on the relationship between science and holiness and on the role of Catholic medicine, to which *La Civiltà Cattolica* sought to provide a response. Salis Seewis chose medical-physiological arguments in his attempt to demonstrate the uncertainty of all hypotheses advanced by doctors, blinded by their trust in science and by their anti-clericalism. The apologetic line, already drafted by *L'Unità Cattolica*, was based on the demonstration of materialist medicine's inability to resolve the issue:

> Rationalist doctors do not act to deny the supernatural because they are induced to do so by progresses in medicine; rather, by refuting it a priori, they sacrifice and forge science in the service of vulgar prejudices. This is a fact. All the theories that we have examined up to here err on the two most essential aspects: the phenomenon aspect,

where they are not able to provide a single identical example with a common nosology, and so they link it to other phenomena that can barely be named as analogous. Regarding the causal aspect, we have witnessed them produce with marvelous frankness causes that are extravagant, false, or insufficient for much minor effects. No science would tolerate such a way of discussing the phenomena; and neither would proper medicine.

(Salis Seewis 1889–1890, 669)

Having set aside, with a certain satisfaction, the "babel confusion of powerless theories" (Salis Seewis 1889–1890, 680) by materialist physicians and having rejected the accusations of quackery advanced by Böens, stating that "charlatans more often dress up as doctors rather than Saints or theologians" (1889–1890, 683), the Jesuit came to support the view that the alleged scientific explanations of medicine could not clarify a divine mystery: the Christly wounds on Louise Lateau's body were the unequivocally visible signs of her holiness.

The last part of this series of articles dealt with visions and apparitions, completing the list of miraculous phenomena. The visions, which were much more frequent compared to the cases of ecstasies and stigmata, were labeled by rationalist physicians (mentioning, among others, the previously introduced Charcot, Warlomont, Charbonnier, and Mantegazza) as hallucinations, as pathological episodes linked to the body rather than to the supernatural. According to Salis Seewis, however, it was necessary to distinguish between proper visions and hallucinations, "so as not to mistake as a supernatural gift what can only be a lesser than natural effect, as it arises from an alteration of fantasy" (1889–1890, 273). But modern medicine had a "vice in its method, that has become too frequent these days: from any similarity found between two phenomena they conclude on their being identical: and they convince themselves that every explanation is good when it serves to suppress the supernatural" (1889–1890, 273). And next to the biblical episodes, there were citations of the recent Marian apparitions at La Salette (1846) and in Lourdes (1858), recognized by the ecclesiastical authority and which had become places of worship and even of miraculous healings through the intercession of Our Lady: thanks to the divine intercession, therapeutic miracles healed the sick bodies of the faithful.

Although it dwelt upon certain phenomena and episodes in particular, the article took on a general significance of fundamental importance within the Catholic press and public opinion, thus deepening the bond between miracle, holiness, and science and making an appeal for the need for a Catholic medicine, against modern science, made of anti-Catholic prejudices and positivist dogmatisms:

Our good readers will have convinced themselves, that it is no lesser a lacking, even in the scientific order, to want to reduce everything to the forces of nature and, in our case, to pathological causes. This, calling it by its name, is a mere crassness of minds enslaved by systematic biases. An open and free mind must embrace with its gaze the Cosmos as it is, with the entire complexity of phenomena and of forces that reveal themselves within it. If a class of phenomena, as it is in fact, reveals a class of agents and actions beyond visible causes, a free mind will understand even this element in the scientific knowledge it has of the Cosmos; and it will not persist in the naïve resolution to accept for good all the inanest explanations, provided that they rule out the preternatural. They say this is science! Science? It is mere faith, not divine, but human: faith in the lessons they had, whilst studying, from their teachers, faith in what is dogmatically stated by the *coryphaei* of rationalism. If only, for the love of God, all men despising and contesting the supernatural could think with their own minds! Many are of great talent; and if they used it with independence, they would undoubtedly rid themselves of many prejudices, which they maintain in pure deference towards the authority of others.

(Salis Seewis 1889–1890, 680)

In conclusion, Salis Seewis' articles represented an interesting example of how Catholic scientific apology worked in the second half of the nineteenth century. The Christian narrative of science involved both the controversy against the lay, positivist, and materialist scientists, and the elaboration of a Catholic science and medicine as a persuasive alternative. *La Civiltà Cattolica* used scientific and medical arguments, besides theological and moral ones, in order to validate the supernatural and divine origin of phenomena like ecstasies, stigmata, and visions, and to criticize the positive scientific method, blind in its trust in the power of science. Overturning the traditional anticlerical interpretation, the Jesuit accused lay scientists of hypocrisy and scientific dogmatism. This apologetic strategy, which became a point of reference in the clerical propaganda, reflected the need to build and reinforce the Catholic presence and its public role in science and medicine—fields more and more significant in Italian and European society, culture, and politics. The case described shows the attempts to reply to the positivist and materialist science, giving an explanation and allowing, at the same time, to safeguard the Catholicism and to use medicine to its advantage.

In this context, in which the biological and medical approaches became central, the body gained a key role in the debate about medicine and divine supernatural in the nineteenth century. As demonstrated especially by the debate on ecstasies and by Louise Lateau's case, the body became symbolically a battlefield between the materialist medicine and the Catholic one. According to Salis Seewis, the bodies of ecstatics and stigmatics showed material signs of sanctity, just like the traditional cult of relics. The appearance on human bodies of these signs of presumed sanctity as well as the inability of medicine in finding natural and pathologic causes gave the Jesuit the chance to underline the limits of science and to state the importance of faith in approaching this kind of phenomena. He concluded that only a Catholic medicine, scientifically authoritative, theologically correct, and morally approved, could study properly the human body and distinguish the corporal signs of supernatural divine origin from the pathological ones. The Jesuit's final aim was to safeguard the role of Catholicism not only in the pastoral care of souls but also in the moral and social management of the body. In the years following Salis Seewis' articles, Catholics continued focusing on the body in order to claim its relationships with divine episodes (not only ecstasies, stigmata, and visions, but also the miraculous healings in Lourdes or the liquefaction of Saint Januarius' blood in Naples), as well as to defend the body of faithful in its material, moral and sexual dimensions from intrusive interventions of the public healthcare, organized and developed in a modern conception, in Italy and Europe, from the end of the nineteenth to the beginning of the twentieth century.

Note

1. Mesmerism (or animal magnetism) took its name from the Austrian physician Franz Anton Mesmer who, in 1778, announced that he had discovered the existence of an impalpable fluid that surrounded and wrapped each body. In finding the cause of diseases, firstly nervous ones, in the imbalances of the fluid's circulation throughout the human body, magnetic therapy intervened to restore balance in the fluid with the skillful action of the magnetizer. During magnetization, the subjects—primarily females—would enter into states of hypnosis and sleepwalk, in the course of which paranormal qualities and faculties, such as foresight, ability to diagnose diseases, glossolalia, and insensitivity to pain could reveal themselves. Mesmerism had been condemned by a scientific committee in 1784, then spread with the French Revolution and later on during the nineteenth century (Darnton 1995; Traetta 2007).

References

Armando, David. 2013. "Spiriti e fluidi: medicina e religione nei documenti del Sant'Uffizio sul magnetismo animale (1840–1856)." In *Médecine et religion: collaborations, compétitions, conflits (XIIe—XXe siècle)*, edited by Maria Pia Donato, Luc Berlivet, Sara Cabibbo, Raimondo Michetti, and Marilyn Nicoud, 194–225. Rome: École Française de Rome.

Boëns, Hubert. 1875. *Louise Lateau, ou les mystères de Bois-d'Haine dévoilés*. Paris: Manceaux.

Bourneville Magloire, Désiré. 1875. *Science et miracle: Louise Lateau, ou la stigmatisée belge*. Paris: Delahaye.

Charbonnier, Nestor. 1875. *Maladies et facultés diverses des mystiques*. Bruxelles: Manceaux.

Darnton, Robert. 1995. *Mesmerism and the End of the Enlightenment in France*. Cambridge: Harvard University Press.

Forno, Mauro. 2012. *Informazione e potere: storia del giornalismo italiano*. Rome/Bari: Laterza.

"I materialisti e le stimmate di Luisa Lateau." 1875. *L'Unità Cattolica* 99, April 27.

Klaniczay, Gàbor. 2013. "Louise Lateau et les stigmatisées du XIXème siècle entre directeurs spirituels, dévots, psychologues et médecins." *Archivio italiano per la storia della pietà* 26: 289–303.

Lefebvre, François. 1870. *Louise Lateau, sa vie, ses stigmates, ses extases*. Louvain: Peeters.

Mantegazza, Paolo. 1887. *Le estasi umane*. Milan: Treves.

Pellicani, Antonio. 1872. *Luisa Lateau, ossia L'estatica dalle stimmate di Bois-D'Haine*. Turin: Tip. Collegio Artigianelli.

Salis Seewis, Francesco. 1888. "Le estasi, la medicina e la Chiesa." *La Civiltà Cattolica* 39 (11): 33–50; 261–281; 400–413. Translated by the author.

Salis Seewis, Francesco. 1889–1890. "Visioni e allucinazioni." *La Civiltà Cattolica* 40 (4): 8–24; 270–281; 669–682. Translated by the author.

Traetta, Luigi. 2007. *La forza che guarisce: Franz Anton Mesmer e la storia del mesmerismo animale*. Bari: Edipuglia.

Traniello, Francesco. 2007. *Religione cattolica e Stato nazionale: dal Risorgimento al secondo dopoguerra*. Bologna: Il Mulino.

Trecco, Lorenzo. 1879. *Avvenimenti meravigliosi antichi e recenti: apparizioni della Salette, di Lourdes, estasi di Luisa Lateau*. Saluzzo: Tip. Lobetti-Bodoni.

Virchow, Rudolf. 1874. *Über Wunder*. Breslau: Morgenstern.

Warlomont, Évariste. 1875. *Louise Lateau. Rapport médical sur la stigmatisée de Bois d'Haine, fait à l'Académie royale de médecine de Belgique au nom d'une commission*. Bruxelles: Mucquardt.

Part II
The Modern Body

4 Making the Body Productive/ Making "the Body" Productive

Steffan Blayney

Cf. Marx, *Capital*, vol. I, chapter XIII and the very interesting analysis in Guerry [sic] and Deleule.

—Michel Foucault

Until recently, the names of François Guéry and Didier Deleule were likely to have registered in the minds of Anglophone readers primarily as the subjects of an obscure and misspelled citation in the pages of a work by a more famous contemporary (Foucault 1991, 221). Despite the endorsement of Michel Foucault (never the most careful of referencers), however, Guéry and Deleule's work has largely been neglected in the intervening years. First published in French in 1972 as *Le Corps productif*, Guéry and Deleule's collaborative essay *The Productive Body* only appeared in a complete English translation for the first time in 2014.

The aforementioned reference—appearing in Foucault's 1975 book *Discipline and Punish*—is intriguing on several levels. It appears at a point in the text—within the famous chapter on "Panopticism"—at which Foucault is seeking to connect the "formation of the disciplinary society" to "a number of broad historical processes—economic, juridico-political and, lastly, scientific—of which it forms a part" (1991, 220). Crucially, argues Foucault, it is impossible to separate the rise of new technologies for the surveillance, ordering, and control of human bodies, which emerged in the eighteenth century, from the growth of capitalism and the expansion of capitalist production in the same period:

> It would not have been possible to solve the problem of the accumulation of men without the growth of an apparatus of production capable of both sustaining them and using them; conversely, the techniques that made the cumulative multiplicity of men useful accelerated the accumulation of capital. At a less general level, the technological mutations of the apparatus of production, the division of labour and the elaboration of the disciplinary techniques sustained an ensemble of very close relations.

(Foucault 1991, 220–221)

Particularly in this context, the reference to Guéry and Deleule is also notable for its proximity to another, weightier citation: Karl Marx's *Capital*. As *The Productive Body*'s translators, Philip Barnard and Stephen Shapiro, note, the reception of Foucault in the Anglophone world has often been characterized by a disavowal of any connection to Marx or Marxism. In some quarters, Foucault has been characterized, or caricatured, as explicitly *anti*-Marxist. Here though—in one of the best-known chapters in perhaps his most read work—Foucault not only explicitly references *Capital* but does so alongside a far lesser-known work by two relatively unknown contemporary philosophers. Part of the attraction of reading Guéry and Deleule today, then, Barnard and Shapiro suggest, is the opportunity it offers to "reopen the walkway between Foucault and Marx for students of both" (2014, 6).

For readers of Foucault in particular, the titular "body" of Guéry and Deleule might provoke particular interest. While Foucault's contribution to understandings of bodies and body history is celebrated, revisiting his work alongside that of Guéry and Deleule can add an extra dimension to our understanding of his ideas and their development. If Foucault's relationship to Marxism has been the subject of controversy, Francois Guéry and Didier Deleule were explicit in drawing their insights directly from Marx.[1] In fact, as Barnard and Shapiro point out, *The Productive Body* can in large part be read as an attempt by the authors to articulate a theory of the social construction of the body implicit in Marx's work.

Elsewhere, I have drawn on the work of Guéry and Deleule to describe the ways in which logics of capitalist efficiency became encoded in medical and scientific models of health and the body in the first decades of the twentieth century (Blayney 2017). In this period, a new "science of work" developed, which aimed explicitly at enhancing the productive powers of the human body. This was a science, in short, which aimed at making the body productive. Here, in addition, I want to reflect more broadly on how the work of Guéry and Deleule might allow us to make "the body" productive as a category of historical analysis, and as a means of understanding and resisting contemporary logics of capitalist hegemony in the present. Before explaining in more detail the thesis developed by Guéry and Deleule and the contributions which I think it can make, however, it is necessary to briefly outline the ways in which historians have approached this elusive category.

Making "The Body" Productive

Over the last three decades, histories of "the body" have proliferated. Some have even been moved to talk of a "somatic turn" in historical scholarship (Cooter 2010, 394). What, though, do historians mean when we talk about "the body"? For many historians, usage of the term has been frustratingly imprecise, such that "discussions of the body are almost incommensurate—and often mutually incomprehensible" across disciplines and specialisms, with "no clear set of structures, behaviours, events, objects, experiences, words and moments to which *body* currently refers" (Bynum 1995, 5). Too often, Kathleen Canning has argued, even when historians invoke "the body" explicitly, the term functions only "to serve as a more fashionable surrogate for sexuality, reproduction or gender without referring to anything specifically identifiable as body, bodily or embodied" (1999, 499).

In one sense, a historical turn to "the body" may seem unnecessary, for it seems self-evident that histories of all kinds have always contained "bodies." We have always been aware that the kings and queens, the soldiers and generals, the workers and bosses that populate our history books inhabited bodies, were subject to bodily constraints, and were vulnerable to the bodily shocks of hunger, disease, violence, and death. As Foucault observed when writing *Discipline and Punish*, historians of medicine and demography had long been interested in "what might seem to be the purely biological base of existence" and its role in historical processes (1991, 25). What characterizes the "somatic turn" in historiography then—a turn which Foucault can himself claim more than a little responsibility for—is less "body history," as Roger Cooter has put it, than "the notion of a historicised body"; the idea that the body itself has a history, which cannot be reduced to any biological or otherwise ahistorical essence (Cooter 2010, 394).

In his work on medicine, imprisonment, and sexuality, Foucault drew attention to the complex social forces and interactions which shape and regulate bodies. "The body," in Foucault's analysis, is not a biological given, but an irreducibly historical phenomenon. To give one example, in his *History of Sexuality*, Foucault described how the Western societies in the eighteenth century witnessed "an explosion of numerous and diverse techniques for achieving the subjugations of bodies and the control of populations" (1990, 140). These techniques, operating both at the level of the individual and of the human species, comprised what Foucault came to call "biopower." In contrast to older forms of power predicated on the threat of death, biopower instead focuses on the promotion of life. Rather than being a negative force, exercised externally—through the repressive apparatuses of the state—biopower is productive, generating norms and standards to which both individual bodies and populations are expected to approximate and exercised primarily through discursive practices which emphasize self-discipline.

From the 1980s, Foucault's insights were taken up by scholars in a number of fields. The body, previously an "absent presence" in the study of human society, suddenly burst into visibility (Shilling 1993, 9). Bryan Turner's 1984 book, *The Body in Society*, strongly influenced by Foucault, drew attention to "the ways in which bodies are produced, cultivated and disciplined in society" (2008, 3). In the same period, feminist, anti-racist, and queer writers and activists were highlighting the links between individual bodies, relationships between bodies, and wider structures of inequality and domination. Uniting these efforts was a conviction that the body is a category that is neither given nor stable but determined by its location in time and space, and its place within structures of power.

Within the discipline of history, a new attention to the body emerging from the 1990s can be placed within a wider challenge to conventional modes of historiography taking place at that time. In this sense, the "somatic turn" can be seen as a part of a wider "cultural" or "linguistic turn," in which previously held assumptions about the stability of objective historical "facts" were overturned by a new focus on language and representation. While historians detailed the social construction of the body and cataloged its changing representations over time, historiography itself was relegated from an authoritative description of past events to simply another participant in the regime of representations, with historians' accounts of the past as socially and culturally determined as any other text (Cooter 2010, 393–394).

Leaving aside the possibility of any return to a now untenable biological essentialism, a few criticisms of this linguistic approach to "the body" of history are worth enumerating. Some historians have argued that the supposed abstraction or reduction of "the body" to discourse leaves little room for the body as a material, embodied presence or site of experience: "the body that eats, that works, that dies, that is afraid" (Bynum 1995, 1). Another set of "materialist" concerns have been raised by those on the left for whom a focus on language and culture has been seen as distracting from the supposedly more important task of class analysis. In this view, a focus on "the body" (often, regrettably, a cipher for race, gender, or sexuality) is seen as providing an alibi for an individualistic politics of identity. Terry Eagleton, representing this position, criticizes Foucault specifically for inaugurating a shift "from production to perversion" and providing theoretical justifications for the "political paralysis" of the Anglo-American academy (1993, 7).

Given this context, it is perhaps unsurprising that the field of labor history—the traditional home of left historians—should have been particularly interested in figuring out the place of "the body" in our histories. In a special edition of the US journal *Labor* in 2007, Ava Baron and Eileen Boris—echoing Joan Scott's famous call for historians to acknowledge gender analysis—set out a case for "the body" as a "useful category" in the history of work and of the working class. Baron and Boris identified three ways in which "the body" might be approached historically: as "discourse and representation," "as a technology of power or site of regulation/discipline," and "as a corporeal or material presence" (2007, 25). More recently, Marjorie Levine-Clark (2015)—whose own work explores the complex relationships between work, the gendered body, law, and welfare—has renewed calls for a greater theoretical engagement by labor historians with "the body."

Taking on this challenge, the problem that presents itself—not only for historians of work but for historians in general—is to develop a meaningful concept of "the body," which can resist collapsing into the play of language and metaphor but without resorting to ahistorical essentialism. In the remainder of this chapter, I will seek to show how the neglected work of Guéry and Deleule might provide a means by which to reintegrate "the body"—as both a discursive and a material fact—into our histories, while avoiding some of the traps outlined above. Before I proceed to a historical case study—exploring scientific approaches to the working body in Britain between the end of the nineteenth century and the Second World War—it will be necessary to briefly outline the content of Guéry and Deleule's joint essay. I will then conclude by suggesting some possible wider implications for the history and politics of "the body" that might have been opened up.

Making the Body Productive

For Francois Guéry and Didier Deleule, the history of the body is necessarily a history of *production*. The body—as the first means by which humans produced their means of subsistence—is the prototypical means of production and, as such, "the privileged instrument from which all developed technology, including machines, may be derived" (Guéry and Deleule 2014, 51).[2] At the same time, it follows, the history of the body is also necessarily a *social* history. Production requires a division of labor, which in turn brings people into social relations. The "biological body" of the individual is thus necessarily brought into a "social body" held together by relations of production.

Guéry and Deleule's social body can be understood in two senses. On one level, the phrase describes an organic combination of bodies, each performing different tasks toward a collective end or ends. Such an organism can be found in Marx's notion of the collective worker: "a productive mechanism whose parts are human beings" (1990, 457). Simultaneously, however, Guéry and Deleule's use of the term indicates a particular ideological conception of the individual body within its social framework.[3] While some form of social body is a prerequisite of any minimally developed society, the precise form which it takes, and the precise relations between the biological and the social, will be historically specific. As new modes of production develop, the relations between producers—the ways in which individual bodies are incorporated into the social—shift accordingly.

Under capitalism, Guéry and Deleule argue, the socialization of the body is accomplished *via* the intercession of a new third body, *the productive body*. For Guéry and Deleule, following Marx, *productivity* refers not simply to a capacity to *produce*, but specifically to the production of surplus-value for a capitalist employer in exchange for a wage. Since, in Marx's terms, the rate of surplus-value is equivalent to the rate of exploitation—the greater the value produced by the worker, the less they receive in wages—the more productive a worker becomes the more they are exploited. "To be a productive worker," as Marx concludes, "is therefore not a piece of luck, but a misfortune" (1990, 644). Under capitalism, Guéry and Deleule argue, "there is a tendency . . . toward the conversion of human material into productive-form" (52). With the rise of modern industry, as work is reorganized in order to obtain the maximum possible surplus, individual bodies are in turn reorganized according to their economic potentials and integrated "within the productive body as elements of production" (52).

The first half of *The Productive Body*, written by Guéry, traces in broad terms the development of the productive body (implicitly in Western Europe) from its origins in the medieval guild to the mechanized factories of the twentieth century. Following Marx's analysis in Part IV of the first volume of *Capital*, Guéry analyzes the transformation of the social body through a series of stages in the development of a capitalist mode of production. The progression from the system of handicraft production (in Marx's terms) through manufacture to large-scale industry entails at each stage, Guéry shows, new relationships between labor, the body and society. With capitalist control over production becoming progressively more dominant, the social body is accordingly reorganized according to the logic of productivity.

The capitalist's desire for an ever greater surplus leads them to pursue ever larger economies of scale, entailing the accumulation of larger numbers of workers together in factories and workshops and the subsequent extension of organization, cooperation, and interdependence. On the one hand therefore, organic bonds between workers are extended and strengthened. The socialization of the labor process under capital, however, is associated with the progressive individuation and isolation of the laborer. Far from harmonizing the biological with the social, the rise of the productive body entails a traumatic split between the worker and the social nature of their work. Thus, as Bernard and Shapiro argue, the making of the productive body is accompanied by the "squeezing out the awareness of the social nature of work, the social body, in favor of a sense of an individualized 'biological body'" (2014, 13).

At the heart of this process, Guéry and Deleule argue, is the separation of intellectual from physical work—the body from the head. The bigger the *collective* worker becomes, the more specialized the task of each individual worker and the more obscure to each the overall scheme of production in which they are embedded. At this stage, the figure of the expert manager—the avatar of capital, or mediator, as Guéry and Deleule put it—appears as the "intellectual element of production" (89), giving organization, purpose, and unity to the fragmented labor process (83). While the capitalist—or their mediator—takes greater control in the organization and planning of the labor process however, the body of the worker is correspondingly reduced to the status of a physical tool, carrying out a specialized, machinelike function. To put it another way, the worker is reduced to their biological, physical body, while capital has "appropriated the intellectual and technical forces of work for itself" (88).

With the development of advanced industrial capitalism, the transformation and fragmentation of the working body is intensified by the introduction of machinery. Here, an increasingly machinelike laborer competes with machinery "just as workers compete with each other in the labor market" (105). Crucially now, the productive body is no longer simply an extension of the collective worker—an organism whose parts are human beings—but a cyborg assemblage of body and machine. Boundaries between living and non-living labor are collapsed. "The productive body ceases to be a biological metaphor" (84) and the biological is reduced to a "body-machine" (97).

Anticipating many of Foucault's arguments about biopower, Guéry and Deleule argue that this ideological ideal of the productive body is in part produced, sustained, and normalized through scientific knowledge and expertise. In Marx's account of the development of capitalism, the introduction of machinery into the labor process had seen not only "the replacement of human force by natural forces," but "the replacement of the rule of thumb by the conscious application of natural science" (1990, 508). As such, argue Guéry and Deleule, in the course of the nineteenth century, the natural sciences had themselves taken on "the role of eminent productive forces, presupposed by production" (84). Just as new technology entered the factory on the terms of the capitalist, however, scientific *knowledge* likewise took its place as "the delegated presence of capital in the process of production" (89). Scientific knowledge under capitalism, it follows, does not serve to benefit the worker but only to increase the amount of surplus-value that can be extracted from them by the capitalist.

What was true of the physical sciences—physics, chemistry, engineering, etc.—Guéry and Deleule argue, was also true of the human sciences. While the twentieth century had seen medical, physiological, and sociological expertise increasingly enter the factory, this had not been done in the interests of workers' well-being, but on the terms of the capitalist. Scientific models of the human body are therefore made in the image of capital, reifying and legitimating "a representation of living beings in which work's production is constitutive of the perceived being" (106).

In Deleule's section of the book, he takes particular aim at the science of psychology, to which he attributes a dual role in the construction of the productive body. On the one hand, the increasingly sophisticated techniques which modern psychology has developed for understanding, measuring, and categorizing individuals have made possible the scientific enhancement of the body's productive capacities: "to adapt the living machine to the dead one, to make the living machine function like a dead machine—without problems, without qualms, and above all without wasting time—to transform the living machine into efficacious motion" (102). Psychological screenings, personality tests, workplace studies, and other psychological interventions have all assisted in fine-tuning individuals and groups to a point of maximum efficiency. At the same time, psychology also has a remedial function, serving to ameliorate the potentially disruptive consequences of capitalism's destruction of preexisting social bonds. As human relations become incorporated within "the overall system of cogs that make up the social mechanism"—as the machine comes to dominate the labor process and the biological body is reduced to the "role of a slave dependent on a 'lifeless mechanism'"—so the "intervention of Psychology will . . . be based on the inevitable need to manage this circuit" (129). As capitalist work becomes ever more alienating, psychological intervention functions "to restore to the subject an alien awareness of his condition" centered on the *ersatz* supplements of "belonging," "group identity," "personality," or "well-being" (131). Importantly, it can be seen, this second function of psychology feeds productively into the first, reducing the potential of resistance and allowing workers to be more efficiently integrated into the productive body.

Here again, Guéry and Deleule's thinking can be seen to chime with that of Foucault in *Discipline and Punish*. In Foucault's account, the rise of industrial capitalism from the eighteenth century was accompanied by a governmentality, which aimed at creating "docile bodies" suited to the demands of production (1991, 135–169). While Guéry and Deleule's argument is in many ways similar, the concept of a *productive* body, as opposed to a docile body, stresses both the centrality of the labor process in the shaping of the body (something Guéry and Deleule consistently emphasize), and the individual body's integration within a larger machine of capitalist production. The focus on productive bodies emphasizes the point—expressed elsewhere by the historian Rudolf Braun—that the docile body is easily converted into "docile capital" (1991, 120). In a final sense, the concept of productivity also neatly captures Foucault's own insight that relations of power are not simply repressive but also themselves *productive*: generative and constitutive of bodies, capacities, and subjects. Capitalism, in Guéry and Deleule's assessment, does not simply "control" our bodies: it makes them *productive* (Barnard and Shapiro 2014, 34).

The Science of Work and the Productive Body

In Western Europe and the United States, between the late nineteenth century and the mid-twentieth, a range of new approaches to the working-class body emerged in which the logics ascribed to the productive body by Guéry and Deleule—*the conversion of human material into productive-form*—were brought to the surface of scientific discourse. With the dual revolutions—industrial and scientific—of the mid-nineteenth century, the electrical motor and the laws of thermodynamics saw the human body remade in terms of "energy" and "work" (Rabinbach 1990). From the end of the nineteenth century, various schemes of "scientific management"—most famously associated with that of Frederick Winslow Taylor—aimed to reorganize the labor process so as to extract the maximum surplus-value from the working body.

In Britain—as I have described elsewhere—the first decades of the twentieth century saw the emergence of a "science of work," distinct from Taylorist scientific management, yet sharing broadly similar motives. Encompassing a range of new "industrial" specialisms—industrial medicine, industrial physiology, industrial psychology, etc.—this new science, I have argued, is best understood as a technology of the productive body. The worker was an object for medical and scientific intervention only insofar as they represented a constituent part of the machinery of industrial labor, while the individual body was, in turn, reimagined as a productive system in microcosm (Blayney 2017).

Late-nineteenth-century British physiology saw the laws of the machine (thermodynamics) applied increasingly explicitly and consistently to the body of the worker. An 1892 textbook characterized the human body authoritatively as a "physical machine," "an engine furnace . . . convert[ing] energy into work" (Starling 1892, 3). Medical and social panics about an epidemic of "fatigue" in the final decades of that century likewise framed the body as an economy of energies, at risk of depletion through unproductive use. Fatigue—the declining capacity of muscle or mind for sustained effort—was understood in terms of reduced "capacity for work" and measured in terms of "output." While concerns about middle- and upper-class "neurasthenics" are well documented, anxiety about working-class fatigue and "industrial neurasthenia," which peaked in the first decades of the twentieth century are, in this context, deserving of more attention (Myers 1920b, 182).

By the time of the First World War, British fatigue research had entered the factory. In contrast to Taylorist scientific management—the domain of the private entrepreneur—this science of work was often backed by the state. The wartime work of the Health of Munition Workers Committee (HMWC), appointed by the British government in 1915 in response to a crisis in armaments production, was continued in peacetime by the Industrial Fatigue Research Board (IFRB), known after 1928 as the Industrial Health Research Board (IHRB). In 1921, these government institutions were joined by the private, not-for-profit National Institute of Industrial Psychology (NIIP). Encompassing a range of expertise, the "work scientists" involved in these institutions' investigations included not only physicians, physiologists, psychologists, but economists, statisticians, employers, trade unionists, and politicians.

The problematic they variously addressed was precisely the question of how the biological body could be incorporated into a social body transformed by mechanization, standardization, and rationalization. As one report put it:

> The mechanization of industrial processes is developing more rapidly than the knowledge of its effects. While much thought and skill have been given to the invention and construction of machines, less attention has been given to the study of their effects on the workers. Thus, whilst the material gains of mechanization . . . are plainly obvious, the strains and stresses experienced by the individuals who operate the machines are often so much less obvious as to be ignored.
>
> (Wyatt and Langdon 1938, iii)

As for Guéry and Deleule, the productive body was conceived of by the science of work as an aggregate of human and mechanical parts. What separated the science of work from Taylorist management systems, its proponents argued, was its systematic consideration of the "human factor" within this assemblage. The labor process, it was argued, could be viewed in terms of "mechanical factors" and "human factors," the former covering the machines and tools used, and the latter describing all the variables that the worker brought to the process. Depending on the kind of work, the proportion of each factor varied: in a completely manual task, the human factor would predominate exclusively, while in a completely mechanized process, it would be absent.

Since the industrial revolution, work scientists argued, attempts to improve productivity had been focused near-entirely on the mechanical side of industry, to the detriment of workers' health and efficiency. "We have perfected the machine in industry," wrote the trade unionist Arthur Pugh, who served on both the NIIP executive committee and the IFRB in the 1920s, "but it has been at the expense of the human factor. . . . We have applied Science to Industry but it has been in relation only to the process of production, not in relation to the human producer" ("The Burlington House Meeting" 1923, 271).

To maximize the productive potential of the population, work scientists argued, it was necessary to study not simply the worker *as a worker*, but "the whole man—his wants, his ideas, and his ideals" (Sorley 1920, 3). The rhetoric of the human factor was used to legitimate calls for increasingly comprehensive medical and psychological control surveillance. As well as experiments on fatigue and working capacity, industrial scientists made wide-ranging recommendations on an expansive array of topics including hours of work, working methods, diet, recreation, and many more topics, and devised complex tests of aptitude, intelligence, and personality.

As in Deleule's characterization of modern psychology, work science's drive to make the body productive was accompanied and enhanced by a complementary focus on consent and harmony. If the worker "is not happy," as one industrial psychologist put it, "he is not likely to be productive" (Bond 1926, 8). For the industrialist Benjamin Seebohm Rowntree, who had been an important early supporter and sponsor of the NIIP, the study of the "human factor in business" was chiefly of importance in tackling problems of industrial unrest, particularly in the tense conditions of British postwar industrial relations (1921, v–ix). The grievances of workers were routinely pathologized, with psychologists advising employers that workplace unrest could be subdued through the "timely application of psychotherapeutic measures (based on the recent developments of abnormal psychology)" (Myers 1920a, 169–170).

Despite work scientists' noble claims to be interested in the "whole man" or in "human nature," the discourse of the human factor in the science of work in practice entailed a radically limited view of what the "human" was. As industrial science designated for itself an ever greater field influence, the worker was correspondingly reduced to a mere element in the industrial process. The human factor, in practical terms, was precisely that: a *factor of production*, to be considered alongside raw materials or machinery. If it was considered a more complex variable, this did not change the fact that the ultimate horizon for its study was the maximization of output and profit. The explicit goal of the science of work was to "turn every ounce of man-power into productive channels" ("Economy" 1931, 551). The more experts talked about the human factor, the more the worker was alienated from their own humanity, reduced to a constituent element in the productive body, to be optimized for maximum efficiency. This was less the humanization of industry than the industrialization of the human.

While historians and sociologists have paid much attention to Taylorist scientific management, the influence of the more respectable science of work has been overlooked. The professional credentials of work scientists, their access to government and institutional support, lent them an authority that allowed their ideas to attain a level of consensus unparalleled by Taylorist efficiency engineers who were easily dismissed as unscientific charlatans or unscrupulous profiteers. If Taylorism, as Harry Braverman has claimed, was "nothing less than the explicit verbalization of the capitalist mode of production" (1998, 60), then the science of work represented its scientific legitimation. The logic of the productive body, latent in the history of capitalism, was written indelibly into mainstream scientific knowledge.

Beyond the Productive Body

In interpreting this historical case study through the lens of *The Productive Body* I have hoped to indicate how a history of making the body productive might open up new ways to make "the body" productive as historians and to resolve some of the contradictions which have divided body historians.

By thinking through the social construction of the body within concrete relations of production, Guéry and Deleule's reading of Marx provides an understanding of the body that is materialist without being essentialist. Moreover, as Barnard and Shapiro have argued, rereading Foucault's work on the body in the light of his connection to Guéry and Deleule allows an interpretation of discursive analysis that complements—not breaks with— a materialist analysis. My suggestion here is not that histories of the body should necessarily be judged according to their adherence to a prescriptive or dogmatic reading of a specific theoretical text or texts, but that the perspectives opened up in this way might provide productive ways for historians to engage with the body anew.

When thinking in structural terms, it is important that we do not flatten difference into a single, homogenized body. When we talk of the disciplinary forces which shape our corporeal reality, it is important that we do not imagine "a universalised body worked upon in a uniform way by surveillance techniques and practices" (Canning 1999, 501). The imposition of discipline and control—the making of docile, useful, and productive bodies—is not a one-sided or linear process. Rather, it is the product of social struggle, often over long periods of time. Finally, in studying discourses we need to be careful not to mistake them for experiences or subjectivities, even while being aware of their mutually constitutive relationships: as much as we focus on the hegemonic discourses and ideologies which shape our bodies, we must also make room for difference, agency, and resistance.

Moreover, in theorizing the history of the body under capitalism, it is also incumbent on us to think beyond it. In *The Productive Body*, scientific knowledge under capitalism is seen as playing an important role in the extraction and appropriation of the body's productive powers. "The corresponding thesis," writes Guéry, "is the idea that socialism is basically the affirmation of the appropriation of the productive sciences by manual workers, which short-circuits capital and contains the productive body within itself so that it can do the bidding of a renewed social body" (92). What Deleule illustrates in his discussion of psychology is that the totalizing logics of the productive body are never fully successful, requiring external interventions to address the alienation and dissatisfaction which are their necessary corollary. The productive body, "constrained as it is to tear life away from living beings in order to reduce them to desirable, machine-like acts, encounters at every step and in all its diverse forms the resistance of life—whether in class struggle, in the form of a resurgence of aspirations for living work, or, in everyday life, as demands for the recognition of alterity" (133).

Today, under the increasingly pervasive influence of what Mark Fisher (2009) has termed "capitalist realism," it has seemingly been impossible to imagine an economic, social, or cultural order—life itself—outside the narrowly defined boundaries of a neoliberal social body. Neoliberalism, as David Harvey has argued, has "become incorporated into the common-sense way many of us interpret, live in, and understand the world" (2007, 3). In such a context, a renewed ability to articulate logics which disrupt or challenge the inevitability of present arrangements is of crucial importance. If the body is a privileged site for the "construction of the inevitable" (Wolf-Meyer 2012, 155), then it is also, as the philosopher John Protevi (2009) has suggested, a point from which to challenge and contest these logics.[4] In this way, too, a historical understanding of the ways that bodies have been made productive makes us responsible for making the body productive in the present.

Notes

1. For a more detailed background on the context in which Guéry and Deleule were writing, their intellectual debts, and political commitments, see Barnard and Shapiro's introduction to *The Productive Body*.
2. For the remainder of the chapter, all page numbers relate to Guéry and Deleule's *The Productive Body* unless otherwise specified.
3. In explaining this doubling of the social body, Guéry and Deleule give the example of Menenius Agrippa's fable of "The Belly and Its Members," in which social relations are mapped onto the relations between parts of the body, though one might also think of the frontispiece to Hobbes' *Leviathan*, in which the body of the Sovereign is depicted as composed of the bodies of his subjects.
4. Cf. the very interesting analysis in Graham Jones (2018).

References

Barnard, Philip, and Stephen Shapiro. 2014. "Editors' Introduction to the English Edition." In *The Productive Body*, edited by François Guéry and Didier Deleule, 1–45. Winchester: Zero Books.

Baron, Ava, and Eileen Boris. 2007. "'The Body' as a Useful Category for History Working-Class History." *Labor* 4 (2): 23–43.

Blayney, Steffan. 2017. "Industrial Fatigue and the Productive Body: The Science of Work in Britain, c. 1900–1918." *Social History of Medicine*, hkx077. https://doi.org/10.1093/shm/hkx077

Bond, Charles J. 1926. *The Human Factor in Industry*. Leicester: W. Thornley & Son.

Braun, Rudolf. 1991. "The 'Docile' Body as an Economic-Industrial Growth Factor." In *Favorites of Fortune: Technology, Growth, and Economic Development since the Industrial Revolution*, edited by David S. Landes, Patrice L. R. Higonnet, and Henry Rosovsky, 120–141. Cambridge, MA: Harvard University Press.

Braverman, Harry. 1998. *Labor and Monopoly Capital: The Degradation of Work in the Twentieth Century*. New York: Monthly Review Press.

"The Burlington House Meeting: Speakers' Addresses." 1923. *Journal of the National Institute of Industrial Psychology* 1 (7): 261–274.

Bynum, Caroline. 1995. "Why All the Fuss about the Body? A Medievalist's Perspective." *Critical Inquiry* 22 (1): 1–33.

Canning, Kathleen. 1999. "The Body as Method? Reflections on the Place of the Body in Gender History." *Gender & History* 11 (3): 499–513.

Cooter, Roger. 2010. "The Turn of the Body: History and the Politics of the Corporeal." *Arbor* 186 (743): 393–405.

Eagleton, Terry. 1993. "It Is Not Quite True That I Have a Body, and Not Quite True That I Am One Either." *London Review of Books* 15 (10): 7–8.

"Economy." 1931. *Industrial Welfare & Personnel Management* 13 (154): 551–552.

Fisher, Mark. 2009. *Capitalist Realism: Is There No Alternative?* Winchester: Zero Books.

Foucault, Michel. 1990. *The History of Sexuality*. Translated by Robert Hurley. Vol. 1. *The Will to Knowledge*. London: Penguin.

Foucault, Michel. 1991. *Discipline and Punish: The Birth of the Prison*. Translated by Allan Sheridan. Harmondsworth: Penguin Books.

Guéry, François, and Didier Deleule. 2014. *The Productive Body*. Translated by Philip Barnard and Stephen Shapiro. Winchester: Zero Books.

Harvey, David. 2007. *A Brief History of Neoliberalism*. Oxford: Oxford University Press.

Jones, Graham. 2018. *The Shock Doctrine of the Left*. Cambridge: Polity.

Levine-Clark, Marjorie. 2015. "*Working Men's Bodies: Work Camps in Britain, 1880–1940* by John Field (Review)." *Labour/Le Travail* 75: 319–320.

Marx, Karl. 1990. *Capital: A Critique of Political Economy*. Vol. 1. London: Penguin.

Myers, Charles S. 1920a. *Mind and Work: The Psychological Factors in Industry and Commerce*. London: University of London Press.

Myers, Charles S. 1920b. "Psychology & Industry." *British Journal of Psychology* 10 (2), March: 177–182.

Protevi, John. 2009. *Political Affect: Connecting the Social and the Somatic*. Minneapolis: University of Minnesota Press.

Rabinbach, Anson. 1990. *The Human Motor: Energy, Fatigue, and the Origins of Modernity*. New York: Basic Books.

Rowntree, Benjamin Seebohm. 1921. *The Human Factor in Business*. London: Longmans, Green & Co.

Shilling, Chris. 1993. *The Body and Social Theory*. London: Sage.

Sorley, William R. 1920. "Some Ethical Aspects of Industry." In *Lectures on Industrial Administration*, edited by Bernard Muscio, 1–12. London: Pitman.

Starling, Ernest Henry. 1892. *Elements of Human Physiology*. London: J. & A. Churchill.

Turner, Bryan W. 2008. *The Body and Society: Explorations in Social Theory*. 3rd edition. London: Sage.

Wolf-Meyer, Matthew J. 2012. *The Slumbering Masses: Sleep, Medicine, and Modern American Life*. Minneapolis: University of Minnesota Press.

Wyatt, S., and James N. Langdon. 1938. *The Machine and the Worker: A Study of Machine Feeding Processes*. Industrial Health Research Board Report 82. London: HMSO.

5 Corpulence, Modernity, and Transcendence in the Early Twentieth Century

Christopher E. Forth

"Oh, look, look!" They spoke in low, scared voices. "Whatever is the matter with her? Why is she so fat?" Such were the questions whispered by the aging but still slim and beautiful elites in Aldous Huxley's *Brave New World*. They had just encountered Linda, who had recently returned from the Savage Reservation where she had been sent years earlier to give birth to her son, John. The reasons for their discomfort were understandable. In a society where eugenic engineering had made it possible to extend youthfulness beyond the biological norm, it stood to reason that they had "never seen a face that was not youthful and taut-skinned, a body that had ceased to be slim and upright." Older than Linda by roughly 20 years, these "moribund sexagenarians had the appearance of childish girls. At 44, Linda seemed, by contrast, a monster of flaccid and distorted senility" (1950, 177).

An exaggeration of contemporary cultural trends for didactic purposes, the future projected in *Brave New World* gathers some of the corporeal fantasies that, in one form or another, have been articulated throughout Western culture. The nightmare that Huxley portrayed was a caricature of the utopian desires he saw manifested all around him: for youth, health, beauty, and performance with few limitations, in a world where illness, ugliness, and aging were coming to be managed by new technologies. As an unsightly sign of age and perhaps sickness—troubling reminders of human finitude but also inescapable facts of organic existence—fatness was but one of the many aspects of "life" that a technological utopia would need to engineer out of existence. This wish for a more or less fat-free world, at least for elites, is hardly novel. Visions of an earthly society or heavenly afterlife inhabited by perfected human forms have inspired health reformers and religious believers for millennia. While the *means* for achieving the ideal body were very different in the past, the future that Huxley feared placed a similar premium on youthfulness and longevity as well as on the eventual elimination of non-normative bodies among the elite.

By exploring the utopian and transcendent yearnings that have informed some of the body cultures of the early twentieth century, this chapter shows that more pronounced ideas about slender and muscular bodies unfolded at the juncture of several developments. Manifested in a variety of domains, from modernist art and literature to modern athletics and high-performance sports to shifting ideas about beauty, health, and aging, anti-fat prejudice accelerated as part of a generalized cultural yearning for forms of transcendence in which frustration with the messy limitations of conventional physicality—as well as an ever-expanding set of challenges posed by the conventions and institutional structures of modernity—encouraged collective dreaming of alternative forms of embodiment. Dreams may have ancient antecedents, but the twentieth century offered the tantalizing technological possibility of bringing them closer to reality. While some of these visions were expressed in the more overtly utopian projects of communism and fascism, this chapter focuses on how mainstream body aspirations reflected these overt dreams of creating perfect worlds. Early twentieth century culture thus crystallized centuries of Western misgivings about fat, fatness, and fattening, marshaling and weaponizing them to the fat phobia of our current world.

Utopia and Transcendence

There is a distinctly modern dimension to fat intolerance, at least when approached in terms of body size and shape. Historians agree that many of the core ingredients of our contemporary anti-fat prejudices had already fallen into place by the time *Brave New World* appeared. By then, bodily ideals within the West had become slenderer than ever before. With scientific advances from the mid-nineteenth century placing food and other commodities within the reach of larger numbers of people, the plumpness that had once symbolized middle-class social privilege lost much of its prestige. As fat bodies became increasingly commonplace, in the social hierarchy they were depressingly "common." With fatness gradually becoming more associated with lower-class and nonwhite bodies, "external signs of wealth [were] displaced into other forms of consumption, [and] the cult of the thin, healthy, sportive, performing and ascetic body dominate[d] in the hierarchy of representations" (Csergo 2009, 27). While the habit of ridiculing fat people seems to have been on the rise throughout the nineteenth century, this tendency was exacerbated by the expanding culture of advertising and mass consumption (Farrell 2011, 3–4). The visual nature of this culture is obvious. Along with European cinema, Hollywood played a memorable role in an ensemble cast. Just as the silver screen projected images of ideal bodies around the world, motion picture fan magazines shared with the masses the reducing diets and fitness regimens of the stars (Addison 2003).

The early twentieth century is a useful site for contemplating our current views of fat. As Georges Vigarello quite rightly states, the "body of the 1920s is quite simply the herald of today's body" (2013, 166). Henceforth, the Western image of corpulent bodies would represent an "aesthetic threat and a health risk" tied to twentieth-century concepts of bodies as consumable objects on display as well as medical problems that would, in time, place burdens on healthcare systems (Vigarello 2013, 148). Having been described as a life-shortening and disfiguring disease since the sixteenth century, "obesity" became even more vocally denounced by doctors as the harbinger of sickness, disability, old age, and death. Demands that people curb their appetites while adopting healthy diet and exercise regimes transformed the body into something that had to be regularly managed through sheer acts of willpower. All of this reflected the paradoxes of a mass society that encourages consumption while simultaneously demanding greater self-control. This self-control, in a further paradox, requires purchasing fitness products and services that are part of the same consumer society credited with producing fatness (Stearns 1997, 60). These trends would develop more fully in the decades to come. With the rise of neoliberalism in the 1970s, as well as the attendant "culture of bulimia" that coupled compulsory consumption with an equally compulsory demand for self-discipline, fatness would become one of the most recognizable emblems of a loss of personal control and a social fall from grace (Guthman 2011, 183). Even if its cultural roots are much deeper than this, our current disgust with fat has its most immediate conditions of possibility in the early twentieth century.

But do these developments adequately address why responses to fat bodies became so visceral and nasty, as if the very existence of the corpulent posed a threat of contamination? Building upon centuries of accumulated misgivings about grease and corpulence, especially as these clashed with evolving ideas about cleanliness, whiteness, and civilization, modern disgust about (and fear of becoming) fat may reflect aspirations that are more utopian and transcendent than usually believed. The word "utopian" is here used in its most basic sense. Ruth Levitas maintains that the "essence of utopia seems to be desire—the desire for a different, better way of being" (2011, 209). She proposes that the sources of what some may call a utopian "impulse" lie in "the human experience of a sense of hunger, loss and lack: a deep sense that something's missing. . . . Everything that reaches to a transformed existence is, in this sense, utopian" (209). In this more or less "existential" definition, utopia is not a concept that depends upon representations of alternative or perfected worlds. Rather it "occurs as an embedded element in a wide range of human practice and culture" (209). This is why Levitas can maintain that "contemporary culture is saturated with utopianism, even (or especially) where there is no figurative representation of an alternative world" (2013, 5).

The family resemblance between utopian and religious wishes is fairly obvious. Both seem to have sources in the ambiguity of embodiment. Much as utopian hope may be grounded in the lived experience of incompleteness—including the universal human grappling with pain, illness, aging, and death—religion's central concept of "transcendence" may also be said to be "anchored in the relative indeterminacy of our embodied existential condition" (Vásquez 2011, 10). Moreover, just as the concept of utopia does not require actual hope for alternative worlds in order to be expressed, transcendence need not be conflated with belief in divine beings or otherworldly realities. Insofar as there may be plausible links between utopian and religious figurations and the kind of magical thinking (Fischler 1996) that structures disgust—an emotion in which, according to Colin McGinn, "we take the measure of the disjunction between how the world actually works and how we would like it to be" (2011, 181)—it is reasonable to see modern anti-fat attitudes as expressing a tendency toward corporeal utopianism and a desire for transcendence. If we define "corporeal utopianism" as culturally inflected wishes for different (and, one assumes, better) forms of embodiment, specifically those that resist the degenerative forces of the environment and are less subject to the exigencies of organic life, then we can see how fat and fatness might emerge as unwelcome reminders of the limits of such wishes. The flight from fat and fatness is an effect of the pursuit of "perfect health," which amounts to a "new utopia," if not a new "eco-bioreligion" (Sfez 1995).

Varieties of corporeal utopianism are evident throughout history, not least in attempts to explore and maximize human perfectibility and in ongoing attempts to extend human life, even to the point of defeating death (Le Dévédec 2015). We see examples of related aspirations in previous centuries. Hopes to overcome the limitations of ordinary embodiment could also be organized collectively. Some argue that Western culture has for centuries manifested a "utopian drive to control the body through the biopower of the state, to make those bodies reproductive, productive, disciplined, fit, homogeneous, normalized, or any other desirable set of traits, whether it is through a direct physical intervention or through the indirect training of citizens to instill self-regulatory practices" (Byers and Stapleton 2015, 5). Others have tracked the rise and fall of a "utopian" attempt to create working bodies that would not succumb to fatigue, a dream buoyed well into the twentieth century by attempts to maximize the machinelike capacities of workers. The science of labor, which achieved its apotheosis in the Fordism and Taylorism of the 1920s and 30s, sought to actualize "the daydream of the late nineteenth-century middle classes—a body without fatigue" (Rabinbach 1992, 44). These machinelike bodies, it was hoped, would be pushed beyond ordinary human capacities so as to never grow tired or require much rest, a fantasy to some extent converted into twentieth-century athletics' dreams of unlimited performance (Hoberman 1992).

Insofar as the ambiguities of embodiment are often experienced on a deeply personal level, not all of these utopian or transcendent desires are entirely reducible to social pressure, as countless personal projects for maximizing health and extending longevity make clear. Dietary reforms and exercise programs have been central to these projects as individuals have sought to live longer, healthier lives. Yet techniques of the self are always enmeshed in social contexts, which means that the management of diet and exercise have typically dovetailed with political and economic agendas. From the mid-nineteenth century onward, nutritional intervention into the diet of workers aimed at promoting efficiency and performance while curtailing the body's natural tendency to dissolution and decay (Rabinbach 1992, 53). It is therefore unsurprising that it was nutritionists who sought to institute a kind of "utopia" in which the "perfect human diet" would be developed to provide "salvation" for all (quoted in Lupton 1996, 7). That the idea of utopia would eventually become individualized with the advent of neoliberalism at the end of the twentieth century does not diminish the persistence of this yearning for experiences that might transcend the limits of ordinary embodiment. Diet and fitness regimes may energize collectives, but they can just as easily offer paths to more personal forms of salvation.

A slippage between ideas about health and "salvation" is commonplace and enduring. It is also quite old. Ancient visitors to the sanctuary of the Greek healing god, Asclepius, left inscriptions indicating that "salvation" (*soteria*) for them resided in the restoration of bodily health on earth rather than in the afterlife (Endsjø 2009, 22). Modern discourses of weight loss and exercise are also replete with images of purification and transcendence, uplifting and overcoming, all of which imply processes of conversion and redemption, whether earthly or spiritual. The British exercise guru Thomas Inch was just one among many who insisted that exercising to lose weight was the key to "physical salvation" (1923, 52). The corpulent physique was thus a "fallen" body in need of redemption. The transcendent aspirations of corporeal utopianism are evident when we consider how often the slender and fit bodies of the twentieth century are photographically captured while airborne or in the act of thrusting upward, momentarily freeing themselves of gravity as they seem to press toward hitherto unimagined heights. With the advent of aviation, humans would literally begin to take flight, and it would not be long before bodies would be even more explicitly likened to streamlined machines efficiently moving through space (Cogdell 2004). To rise above all manner of constraints—the earth, animality, primitivity, tradition, history, aging, and even death itself: such are the somatechnical hopes that fueled the bodily dreams and ideals of the modern world. Having come to be more closely linked to greasy and filthy substances, animalistic habits, and lower-class as well as nonwhite populations (Forth 2012a, 2012b), fat, fatness, and fattening were readily cast as obstacles to be overcome on the path to regeneration and transcendence.

Modern Transcendence

Insistence on the modernity of our present-day fat prejudices is widespread and, in some respects, well-founded. There is ample evidence that an already limited tolerance for fat and fatness diminished at an uneven pace throughout the modern era, even if there is some lack of consensus on what constitutes "modernity" and when this supposedly distinct period began. Without delving into the quandary created by questions of definition and periodization, it is tempting to transpose social theorist Zygmunt Bauman's (2000) contrast between "heavy" and "light" modernity to the history of body ideals. Our current phase of lipophobia, which emerged in full force during the 1970s, does seem to coincide with the end of an era characterized by territorial expansion, mining, industrialization, large machines, and "hardware" of every sort. As opposed to this "heavy" modernity that had been developing since the age of empire and industrialization, our present moment manifests a clear preference for lightness, movement, fluidity, and instantaneity. "Giant industrial plants and corpulent bodies have had their day," Bauman remarks. "[O]nce they bore witness to their owners' power and might; now they presage defeat in the next round of acceleration and so signal impotence" (2000, 128).

There is something appealing about this explanation. It is true that what Bauman calls "light modernity" places a premium on movement, speed, and cleanliness, all of which have been contrasted to the heaviness of tradition, history, and, of course, the body itself. Yet speed, fluidity, and ephemerality have been part of the experience of urban modernity before the poet Charles Baudelaire made a note of them in the early 1860s. Moreover, as we have seen, the heavy bodies of elites never offered unequivocal evidence of status and power. It was precisely during the imperial era that the corpulence of some indigenous and colonized peoples became a reliable countertype to an emergent ideal of "civilized" moderation and muscularity. Distinctions between "heavy" and "light" modernity can be only unevenly mapped onto fat and thin bodily ideals.

It is possible to approach the relationship between fatness and modernity in other ways. A commonsense way of thinking about the modern, at least in temporal terms, is to assume a radical break with the past and a futural orientation for our thought and actions. But the modern is also something that is lived. Susan Stanford Friedman proposes a working definition of "modernity" that takes experience as its core: "The velocity, acceleration, and dynamism of shattering change across a wide spectrum of societal institutions are key components of modernity as I see it—change that interweaves the cultural, economic, political, religious, familial, sexual, aesthetic, technological, and so forth, and can move in both utopic and dystopic directions" (2006, 433). What is not often acknowledged in views of modernity-as-novelty is the extent to which models from the distant past may be recycled as examples for living in the present and future. This reaching backwards is often done with an eye toward overcoming aspects of modern life that strike observers as unhealthy or immoral. The persistence of the Spartan mirage in Western culture is a case in point, as are related claims that our ancient or even prehistoric ancestors held the keys to healthy and moral living.

The historian Roger Griffin has sought to account for this strange braiding of old and new in many forms of modernism. Griffin claims that lurking behind what many scholars see as a bewildering array of modernisms—be they aesthetic or social and political in nature—is "a common matrix" that may be "usefully seen as the search for transcendence and regeneration" that is itself a variation of the archaic human myth of rebirth, or what he calls "palingenesis" (2007, 39). The "New Man" often imagined in modern times is quite often an implicitly male being requiring some rejuvenated form of "New Woman" as his partner and breeder. Thus the regeneration promised by many modernist social programs often entails a restoration of traditional gender roles—the (re) creation of "real" men and women—in a social order that believes it has jettisoned the degenerative elements of modernity while still remaining recognizably modern. This is evident in some of the most self-consciously utopian political and social movements of the twentieth century. Although there is no space to investigate them here, both the *homo sovieticus* imagined in Russia after 1917 and the "anthropological revolution" proposed by fascist theorists in Italy may be viewed as pronounced extensions of this deeply ingrained modern response to modernity's excesses (Clark 1993, 33–50; Gentile 2004). Revolution, regeneration, and rejuvenation often presuppose a future that has been reconnected to the most healthy and admirable models of the past. In this sense, as Lynda Nead proposes, modernity may be "imagined as pleated or crumpled time, drawing together past, present and future into constant and unexpected relations and the product of a multiplicity of historical eras" (2000, 8).

Expressing "the desire for a different, better way of being," a range of broadly utopian wishes were widespread during the early twentieth century, not least as responses to the experience of modernity as crisis and discontinuity. The claim that Western societies at the end of the nineteenth century saw themselves in the throes of decadence and degeneration is irrefutable, as is the fact that many individuals and groups engaged in projects aiming at a regeneration of one form or other. Regeneration implied rejuvenation and thus an attempt to recapture youthful energy and beauty in the face of processes of decline. In the United States, for instance, "a widespread yearning for regeneration—for rebirth that was variously spiritual, moral, and physical—penetrated public life, inspiring movements and policies that formed the foundation for American society in the twentieth century" (Lears 2009, 1). It is not coincidental that the body would form the basis for all manner of regenerations, in the United States and elsewhere. "As the public world outside the self becomes diffuse, distant, governed by institutions we cannot control or even influence, the body remains important as an arena we can actually control—or we think we can. It becomes a domain of self-expression, a field for developing one's own set of cultural meanings, and a source, quite naturally, of anxiety" (Lears 1989, 63). If the body became so central to twentieth and twenty-first century culture, it is partly because the often-disorienting experience of modernity transformed it into a deceptively stable site for meaning and transformation, personally as well as collectively.

A longing for rebirth or transcendence, which has often been framed as a kind of salvation from a decadent or degenerate world, is implicit in many forms of the modern. Insofar as the body became the locus of personal and social transformation, it was here that tensions between degeneration and regeneration were played out, whether in esoteric and countercultural philosophies or within more conventional scientific frameworks (Griffin 2007). For many, the apotheosis of the catastrophe of modernity was the First World War, which played a significant role in promoting the celebration of new bodily ideals that proliferated in the following decades. Wounded and disfigured soldiers returned from the trenches as living embodiments of the fears of the able-bodied. The restoration of corporeal wholeness after the war was accompanied by a "spiritual" yearning that, whether expressed through conventional Judeo-Christian categories or any number of "pagan" ideas and images, expressed desires for something more than the grossly material (Carden-Coyne 2009). This yearning was for a kind of disembodied "will" that nevertheless required the performance of the body in order to actualize itself, instantiating the perennial and paradoxical tendency to employ the body to transcend corporeality.

A rather explicit denigration of fat, understood literally as well as metaphorically, is evident in certain forms of aesthetic modernism, which may be seen as "the expressive dimension of modernity" (Friedman 2006, 432). Although "modernism" is itself a loose and imprecise category, much of the painting and architecture as well as the poetry and literature that merits this label displays contempt for the ornate, superfluous, and "feminine," positing instead forms and lines that have been purified, hardened, and masculinized. The Italian Futurists famously epitomized this virile move to purge poetic language of its Victorian superfluity, cutting away "the flab of adjectives and other emasculating parts of speech" (Segal 1998, 2). A similar modernist impulse to eliminate the superfluous and inefficient took place a few decades later in the cultural rhetoric surrounding "streamlining," a concept developed in industrial design and extended to thinking about the size, shape, and eugenic worth of individual bodies. Like an animal or object moving swiftly through a stream of fluid, cars, buses, airplanes, and even human bodies were to be engineered so as to maximize efficiency while minimizing all that might cause friction or the backward tug of "drag" (Cogdell 2004).

Despite its claims to have broken with the past and dispensed with history, modern art has often raided antiquity as well as the non-Western world for its models. After all, the Greeks and Romans seemed to worship muscular hardness as well, and modern notions of beauty have not completely dispensed with classical antecedents. Historian Ana Carden-Coyne (2009) is perhaps the most authoritative guide to the physical and symbolic reconstruction of bodies after the First World War. With the Great War sometimes imagined as a collective sacrifice that would "purge the world of its moral miasma" (124) classical aesthetics played an important role in the cleansing process that aimed at the elevation of bodies as well as morals. Such uses of Classicism are examples of a "cultural nostalgia," defined as "partly a longing for, or an idealizing of, the past, and partly a need to make productive use of the past through cultural practices" (35). In the 1920s and 30s, slenderness became "the visible display of modern 'ultra-civilization'" (249) to the extent that swollen and misshapen bodies were increasingly described as throwbacks to earlier ways of life. Classical models that had been put to effective use in the physical culture movement, and which had gained momentum from the 1880s onward, returned with renewed vigor after the war as "utopian visions of the classical past and the modern future" (263) merged. Statues and monuments commemorating the carnage made use of classical motifs to project images of "masculine beauty frozen in a timeless vortex" offering "the fantasy of eternal renewal, and the avoidance of death" (155). The classical style's formal sterility worked well alongside some versions of the modernist style, making it seem "clean" and thus available for new conceptions of hygiene. Even if the more hedonistic postwar culture promoted comfort and pleasure over sacrifice, neoclassical ideals remained as an ingredient in the demonization of fat that followed (Addison 2003, 10–12).

Whether in the form of avant-garde experiments or neoclassical revivals, modern ideas about the body were vernacularized in—perhaps even abetted by—emerging ideals about the sportive and fit body. In athletics and other forms of physical culture, the aim was less to transcend the body per se than to create one that offered the appearance, and even the sensation, of transcendence. This is why some enlisted stock images of the human body as a kind of machine while downplaying its troubling organic qualities. In this way, the ideal body could be imagined as streamlined and efficient, much like the vehicles and appliances being produced by industry. This forward-looking vision of machinelike bodies presented fatness as a form of "drag" and "waste" that diminished speed, efficiency, and productivity. "Streamline your figure" was the advice of Sylvia of Hollywood, fitness trainer of the stars. Since weight gain was partly linked to undigested food and other residues, one had to purge the system by way of colonic irrigation before beginning any kind of weight-loss plan. "It's like changing the oil in a car," Sylvia explained; "they drain out the old worn oil and sediment before putting in the new" (1939, 31). As effects of "pleated or crumpled time," modern concepts of hygiene, as well as emerging ideals of hairlessness, were based at once on the sanitized "skin" of modern vehicles and the smooth and sterile contours of classical statuary (Carden-Coyne 2009, 256). Even classical ballet displayed bodies that evoked "the arresting beauty of a finished airplane, where every detail, as well as the general effect, expresses one supreme object—that of speed" (André Levinson, quoted in Karthas 2015, 201). A slender body was now a modern body, as readers were reminded even in magazine advertisements. As a 1932 ad for Sun-Maid proclaimed, the fact that raisins burn fat "will mean much in the lives of modern women who wish to remain modern" (Parkin 2007, 174).

In their efforts to whip ordinary citizens into shape for the greater good, proponents of physical culture were animated by "a problem of *too much body*, or at least too much of the wrong kind of body. . . . [They] saw their mission as that of reining in the overwhelming presence of a body in excess" (Cowan 2008, 113). As perhaps the most conspicuous sign of this "excessive" flesh, fatness was one of the conditions that physical culturists and sporting enthusiasts insisted upon overcoming. The explosion of skiing culture in the twentieth century captured some of these aspirations. The German enthusiast Carl Luther claimed that Alpine skiing was particularly attractive to modern people "because we live faster and must demonstrate greater resistance—because we do not wish to age, but rather to remain young, fresh, and slender" (quoted in Denning 2015, 76). Some even propose that modernist culture, broadly construed, is informed by an "anorexic aesthetic" predicated on a rejection of all that the "feminine" seems to represent in Western culture. This is a chain of associations that we have encountered repeatedly in previous chapters: "Femininity is interchangeable with softness; softness is represented by bodily fat; and all of these things—femininity, softness, and fat—are 'disgusting.' . . . Anorexia is a reaction to pervasive cultural symbols related to femininity" (Heywood 1996, 68). If the skeletal appearance of anorexic bodies is one (albeit extreme) response to the "femininity" of corpulence, we must remember that bone is not the only "other" of fat. The hard muscles promoted by physical culture are a central leitmotif of modernity as well, and many who have fled the seemingly corrupting softness of fat have sought refuge within their deceptively reassuring firmness.

Amid all of these changes, the slippage between animalization and racialization cannot be ignored. As we have seen, the colonial world played an essential role in throwing into relief the kinds of regenerated bodies that white Westerners aspired to possess. By the early twentieth century, it was taken for granted that a preference for fatness, whether in oneself or in others, reflected a kind of primitive desire that was out of step with the purportedly loftier aesthetic sensibilities of the Western world. This is why authors like Henry Finck could claim how "savage" it was when supposedly "civilized" people manifested a preference for fleshy bodies. When the demand for slenderness became more pronounced in the 1920s, by which time physical reformers were promoting a transnational rejuvenation of Western civilization, Finck channeled his racialized disgust for fat into a weight-loss book entitled *Girth Control*. Reminding readers of those places in the world "where beauty means fat," he pointedly compared certain "American women of our day" to the "much admired dusky wonders of obesity" overseas (1923, 2–4).

The continuing animalization of "backward" colonial peoples only served to strengthen the "civilized" white person's shaky claim to represent the truly human. So common was this animalization that Frantz Fanon felt compelled to address it decades later. "When the colonist speaks of the colonized he uses zoological terms," Fanon pointed out, a practice that typically evoked "obese bodies that no longer resemble anything" (2002, 45). Tacitly informing the racialization of fatness was the closely related problem of fattening, which evoked perennial misgivings about docile animals fed for the benefit of others. Raising the prospect of becoming fattened and subordinate "beasts," like certain people overseas were said to be, was one way of shaming whites into weight-loss regimes. As French fitness guru Georges Hébert declared, only "certain sedentary domestic animals and gluttons present traces of adiposity" as well as those "oriental peoples" whose taste for fat female bodies evinces "a complete aberration of the aesthetic sense" (1921, 114). Aside from signifying disgusting aesthetic and sexual tastes, fattening remained an issue of gendered power relations. Drawing direct analogies between "the obese man and the animal being fattened for the kill [*l'animal à l'engrais*]," the physician Francis Heckel described the fat man as "a monster ill-adapted to his human function" (1930, 28). Insofar as the act of fattening constitutes beauty only among pigs, sheep, and cows, it was completely at odds with masculinity. "Fat devirilizes and emasculates" (Heckel 1930, 28). Far from being consigned to the dustbin of history, ancient tropes connecting fat with animality, docility, and femininity continued to structure modern perceptions of bodies well into the twentieth century, and beyond.

Conclusion

Extending and reworking aspects of a fat imaginary whose sources are traceable to antiquity, the early twentieth century promoted the "civilized" white body, the hallmarks of which are the clean, smooth, and light, the efficiently quantifiable and predictable, with traces of the organic or animal removed or pushed out of sight and mind. It is not an exaggeration to treat such developments as broadly "utopian" or to suggest that they have been pursued with an almost "religious" fervor. To imagine bodies as efficient, streamlined, and machinelike is to indulge in a fantasy of temporary transcendence of the messy realities of organic life and of the fragile creatureliness that humans share with non-human animals. Alongside these ideals, or implicit within them, are closely related fantasies of purity—of food, hygiene, sexuality, race, etc. The violence with which modern disgust at fat is often manifested seems aimed at driving it out of existence, as if affirming the claim that the "aim of utopias, to a greater or lesser extent, is to eliminate real people" (Carey 1999, xii).

References

Addison, Heather. 2003. *Hollywood and the Rise of Physical Culture*. New York: Routledge.

Bauman, Zygmunt. 2000. *Liquid Modernity*. Cambridge: Polity.

Byers, Andrew, and Patricia Stapleton. 2015. "Introduction." In *Biopolitics and Utopia: An Interdisciplinary Reader*, edited by Andrew Byers and Patricia Stapleton, 1–9. New York: Palgrave.

Carden-Coyne, Ana. 2009. *Reconstructing the Body: Classicism, Modernism, and the First World War*. Oxford: Oxford University Press.

Carey, John. 1999. *The Faber Book of Utopias*. London: Faber and Faber.

Clark, Toby. 1993. "The 'New Man's' Body: A Motif in Early Soviet Culture." In *Art of the Soviets: Painting, Sculpture and Architecture in a One-Party State, 1917–1992*, edited by M. C. Bown and B. Taylor, 33–50. Manchester: Manchester University Press.

Cogdell, Christina. 2004. *Eugenic Design: Streamlining America in the 1930s*. Philadelphia: University of Pennsylvania Press.

Cowan, Michael. 2008. *Cult of the Will: Nervousness and German Modernity*. University Park: Pennsylvania State University Press.

Csergo, Julia. 2009. "Quand l'obésité des gourmands devient une maladie de civilisation: Le discours médicale, 1850–1930." In *Trop gros? L'obésité et ses représentations*, edited by Julia Csergo, 14–32. Paris: Autrement.

Denning, Andrew. 2015. *Skiing into Modernity: A Cultural and Environmental History*. Berkeley: University of California Press.

Endsjø, Dag Øistein. 2009. *Greek Resurrection Beliefs and the Success of Christianity*. London: Palgrave.

Fanon, Frantz. 2002. *Les damnés de la terre*. Paris: La Découverte.

Farrell, Amy Erdman. 2011. *Fat Shame: Stigma and the Fat Body in American Culture*. New York: New York University Press.

Finck, Henry T. 1923. *Girth Control: For Womanly Beauty, Manly Strength, Health, and a Long Life for Everybody*. New York: Harper & Brothers.

Fischler, Claude. 1996. "Pensée magique et utopie dans la science." In *Pensée magique et alimentation aujourd'hui*, edited by Claude Fischler, 1–17. Paris: Les Cahiers de l'OCHA.

Forth, Christopher E. 2012a. "Fat, Desire, and Disgust in the Colonial Imagination." *History Workshop Journal* 73 (1): 211–239.

Forth, Christopher E. 2012b. "Melting Moments: The Greasy Sources of Modern Perceptions of Fat." *Cultural History* 1 (1): 83–107.

Friedman, Susan Stanford. 2006. "Periodizing Modernism: Postcolonial Modernities and the Space/Time Borders of Modernist Studies." *Modernism/Modernity* 13 (3): 425–443.

Gentile, Emilio. 2004. "L'homme nouveau' du fascisme: Réflexions sur une expérience de révolution anthropologique." In *L'homme nouveau dans l'Europe fasciste (1922–1945): Entre dictature et totalitarisme*, edited by M.-A. Matard-Bonucci and P. Milza, 35–63. Paris: Fayard.

Griffin, Roger. 2007. *Modernism and Fascism: The Sense of a Beginning under Mussolini and Hitler*. Basingstoke: Palgrave.

Guthman, Julie. 2011. *Weighing In: Obesity, Food Justice, and the Limits of Capitalism*. Berkeley: University of California Press.

Hébert, Georges. 1921. *Muscle et beauté plastique: l'éducation physique feminine*. Paris: Librairie Vuibert.

Heckel, Francis. 1930. *Maigrir: pourquoi? comment?* Paris: La Renaissance du livre.

Heywood, Leslie. 1996. *Dedication to Hunger: The Anorexic Aesthetic in Modern Culture*. Berkeley: University of California Press.

Hoberman, John. 1992. *Mortal Engines: The Science of Performance and the Dehumanization of Sport*. New York: The Free Press.

Huxley, Aldous. 1950. *Brave New World*. New York: Harper & Brothers.

Inch, Thomas. 1923. *Inch on Fitness*. London: George Newnes.

Karthas, Ilyana. 2015. *When Ballet became French: Modern Ballet and the Cultural Politics of France, 1909–1939*. Montreal: McGill-Queens University Press.

Lears, T. J. Jackson. 1989. "American Advertising and the Reconstruction of the Body, 1880–1930." In *Fitness in American Culture: Images of Health, Sport, and the Body, 1830–1940*, edited by Kathryn Grover, 47–66. Amherst: University of Massachusetts Press.

Lears, T. J. Jackson. 2009. *Rebirth of a Nation: The Making of Modern America, 1877–1920*. New York: HarperCollins.

Le Dévédec, Nicolas. 2015. *La société de l'amélioration. La perfectibilité humaine des Lumières au transhumanisme*. Montreal: Liber.

Levitas, Ruth. 2011. *The Concept of Utopia*. Oxford: Peter Lang.

Levitas, Ruth. 2013. *Utopia as Method: The Imaginary Reconstitution of Society*. Basingstoke: Palgrave.

Lupton, Deborah. 1996. *Food, the Body and the Self*. London: Sage.

McGinn, Colin. 2011. *The Meaning of Disgust*. Oxford: Oxford University Press.

Nead, Lynda. 2000. *Victorian Babylon: People, Streets and Images in Nineteenth-Century London*. New Haven, CT: Yale University Press.

Parkin, Katherine J. 2007. *Food Is Love: Advertising and Gender Roles in Modern America*. Philadelphia: University of Pennsylvania Press.

Rabinbach, Anson. 1992. *The Human Motor: Energy, Fatigue, and the Origins of Modernity*. Princeton: Princeton University Press.

Segal, Harold B. 1998. *Body Ascendant: Modernism and the Physical Imperative*. Baltimore: Johns Hopkins University Press.

Sfez, Lucien. 1995. *La santé parfait. Critique d'une nouvelle utopie*. Paris: Seuil.

Stearns, Peter N. 1997. *Fat History: Bodies and Beauty in the Modern West*. New York: New York University Press.

Sylvia of Hollywood. 1939. *Streamline Your Figure*. New York: McFadden Book Co.

Vásquez, Manuel A. 2011. *More Than Belief: A Materialist Theory of Religion*. New York: Oxford University Press.

Vigarello, Georges. 2013. *The Metamorphoses of Fat: A History of Obesity*. Translated by C. Jon Delogu. New York: Columbia University Press.

Part III
The Visual Body

6   The Visual Politics of the Body in Germany Between the Two World Wars

Claude Lacroix

Between the two World Wars, the human body became one of the ideological battlegrounds in Germany where complex social, cultural, and political forces clashed. The extreme forms these confrontations took are best epitomized, as we will see, by two statements: one made by Dadaist Richard Huelsenbeck months before the end of First World War; the other by Adolf Hitler at the opening of the Great German Art Exhibition in 1937. Conflicting world views were also embodied in the arts and the media. After observing the horrors of war as soldiers, artists such as George Grosz, Otto Dix, and Max Beckmann depicted the tragic consequences of war on the body; so did Ernst Friedrich in his book *Krieg dem Kriege! War against War! Guerre à la Guerre! Oorlog An Den Oorlog!*, published in 1924. That same year, photographs of athletic bodies appeared in Hans Surén's *Der Mensch und die Sonne* (*Man and Sunlight*), one of several publications in the 1920s that equated beauty with health, gymnastics, and nudism. Films such as *Wege zu Kraft und Schönheit* (*Ways to Strength and Beauty*; 1925), directed by Wilhelm Prager and Nicholas Kaufmann, and *Olympia* (1938), directed by Leni Riefenstahl, also greatly contributed to the popular obsession with physical beauty. Ana Carden-Coyne interprets this cult of the body as "an antidote to the physical and emotional suffering of the war . . . a riposte for the loss of life, limb and mind," a form of "liberation" (2009, 21). However, near the end of the interwar period, two major art shows were organized by the Nazis: the Great German Art Exhibition and *Degenerate Art*—a vilification of modern art that included works by Grosz, Dix, and Beckmann, among others. Given the context, can idealization of the body still be perceived as some kind of liberation and remedy to the ills of war?

When Huelsenbeck returned to Berlin in early 1917, he found people impoverished, hungry, and desperate in their anticipation of defeat, beggars and injured soldiers on the streets, the country on the verge of a social revolution. At the first Dada evening held in Berlin on 12 April 1918, he read a manifesto in which he declared:

> Art . . . depends on the time in which it lives. . . . The highest art . . . allows itself to be noticeably shattered by last week's explosions,

which is forever trying to collect itself after the shock of recent days. The best and most challenging artists will be those who every hour snatch the tatters of their bodies out of the turbulent whirl of life, who, with bleeding hands and hearts, hold fast to the intelligence of their time.

(Huelsenbeck 1993, 267)

Although Huelsenbeck had volunteered for military service when the war began and served for several months, he was not sent to the front and was released from service because of neuralgia. He became increasingly opposed to the strong German nationalist feelings and to war, which clearly reflects in the analogies he makes between art and the shock of an explosion, and artists and torn bodies. War had caused death and devastation on an unprecedented scale: an estimated two million German soldiers were killed or went missing; four million were wounded. As pointed out by Carol Poore, "in the chaotic immediate postwar years, progressive and leftist artists and writers turned to the depictions of disability in their search for convincing ways to denounce German militarism and capitalism" (2007, 20).

Grosz, who served six months in the army in November 1914 and four months again in 1917, was thereafter driven by his traumatic experiences to rally against war. He later explained that his "drawings expressed [his] despair, hate and disillusionment [as he] drew soldiers without noses; war cripples" (1946, 146–147). One example of such work is *Deutschland, Deutschland über alles, über alles in der Welt! (Diese Kriegsverletzten)* [*Germany, Germany over All, Over Everything in the World! (These War Casualties)*] (see Figure 6.1). It takes its title from the German national anthem playing on a gramophone while disabled and destitute war veterans with crutches and scarred faces beg. One of them, who has both hands and lower legs amputated, has removed his prostheses to exhibit his leg stumps. His eyepatch indicates that he has also lost an eye in combat. His mutilated body contrasts highly with the fat well-dressed capitalist sitting in the center, who, having benefited from war hostilities, stands for a corrupted and immoral German society. Given that he hands them out money, the drawing is a bitter social caricature in which the mutilated officers are depicted at once as victims and grotesque accomplices in what Grosz called insane "mass slaughter" (1946, 161).

At the outbreak of war, Beckmann was already established with some success as an artist. He volunteered as a medical orderly in the Medical Corps and was posted in a field hospital. Deeply touched by what he saw there, he suffered a nervous breakdown in 1915 and was released from the army. The traumatic experiences of war shaped his view of the world and his art. His commitment to showing the brutal reality of war and "expos[ing] the ghastly cry of the poor disillusioned people" (quoted in Long 1993, 151) can be seen in *Nachhauseweg (The Way Home)* (see

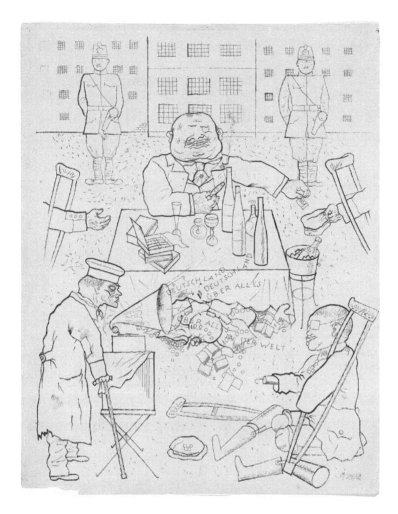

Figure 6.1 George Grosz (1893–1959), *Deutschland, Deutschland über alles, über alles in der Welt! (Diese Kriegsverletzten)* [*Germany, Germany over All, Over Everything in the World! (These War Casualties)*] (circa 1920). Reed pen and India ink on paper, 53 × 41.3 cm

Figure 6.2), from a portfolio of ten large lithographs entitled *Die Hölle* (*HELL*). The night scene features Beckmann himself in a suit and bowler, who has encountered a disfigured veteran. He grasps his arm-stump with one hand to guide him and points out "the way home" with the other. As the war cripple stands under the light of the street lamp, the viewer is confronted with his face: half of it has been blown away along with

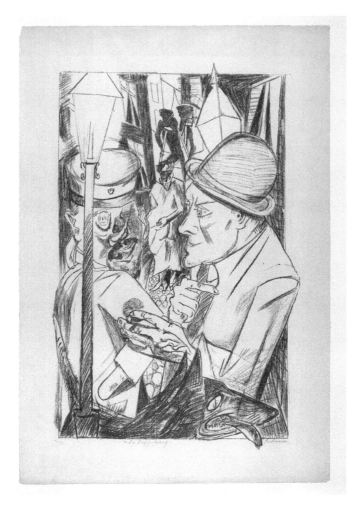

Figure 6.2 Max Beckmann (1884–1950), *The Way Home [Nachhauseweg]*, plate 2 from the portfolio *HELL [Die Hölle]* (1919). Lithograph, printed in black, composition: 29 1/4 × 19 1/16" (74.3 × 48.5 cm); sheet: 34 1/4 × 24" (87 × 61 cm). Abby Aldrich Rockefeller Fund. (468.1949)

his nose and, judging from his remaining eye, he is blind. Further up the street, two more veterans on crutches hobble in the dark.

Dix was a student at the School of Art in Dresden when the war broke out. He spent four years as a machine gunner in the trenches; he was wounded several times and discharged of service. The war experience modified his outlook considerably and made him fiercely anti-militaristic.

He stated that he wanted "to present war objectively . . . and the consequences of war" (Löffler 1982, 70), which he did in *Kriegskrüppel (45% erwerbsfähig!)* [*War Cripples (45% Fit for Work!)*] (see Figure 6.3). Four amputees parade the street; all have one or both legs amputated, two of them an arm, and one is limbless. Except for the man in a wheelchair, whose dark glasses indicate that he is blind, they are outfitted with prostheses: a simple hook, wooden legs, and, in the case of the soldier pushing the wheelchair, sophisticated prostheses represented by the dotted lines and articulations with springs drawn on the side of his clothes along his arm and leg. Two of the veterans have suffered severe facial injuries: one has lost his nose, teeth show through his cheek, the side of his face is badly scarred, and his ear is gone; the other has a steel jaw fixed to his cheekbone with a spring, a kind of hearing trumpet, and what appears to be a glass eye. He must have lost the ability to speak for he seems to communicate by pointing at letters on an alphabet card hanging from his neck (Reily, Panhan, and Tupinambá 2009, 220). As for the man whose head and arm tremble: he is a traumatized soldier, a victim of shell shock. The painting's subtitle, *45% Fit for Work!*, is a satirical reference to the way veteran pension benefits were determined depending on the degree of physical injuries and disabilities one had (Murray 2012, 22). Conrad Felixmüller reported

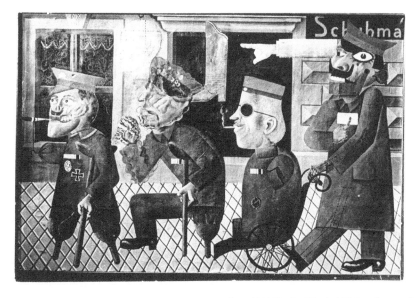

Figure 6.3 Otto Dix (1891–1969), *War Cripples (45% Fit for Work!)* [*Kriegskrüppel (45% erwerbsfähig!)*] (1920). Oil on canvas, 150 × 200 cm. Inv.-Nr. 21/46. Believed destroyed in 1942

Photo from the "Entartete Kunst" exhibition (1937). Bayerische Staatsbibliothek. © Estate of Otto Dix/SOCAN (2018). © ARS, NY. Photo Credit: bpk Bildagentur/Art Resource, NY.

that Dix also subtitled it *Four of These Don't Add Up to a Whole Man* (Eberle 1985, 44), which further emphasizes that artificial limbs can never repair the disabled to the full capacities they once had.

Writing about Beckmann's *HELL* in 1920, Paul Schmidt noted that "the first impression . . . is that of a terrible shock" (1993, 152). As much as the images by Beckmann, Grosz, and Dix are shocking, they cannot compare to the photos that the anarchist and pacifist Ernst Friedrich printed in a book titled *War against War!* (1924), some of which he displayed in the front window of his Anti-War Museum in Berlin: devastated battlefields, destroyed buildings, starving civilians, amputated soldiers, army executions, and piles of dead bodies make dreadfully real pictures. Usually found in military and medical archives, such documents were deemed unacceptable by government censors and held from publication for being too shocking or damaging to the public's morale and support. When Friedrich published these atrocities of war in juxtaposition with sarcastic captions in four languages (German, English, French, and Dutch), inspired by patriotic and military rhetoric about "the field of Honour" and "heroic death," he intended to horrify, demoralize, and shock readers into rejecting all future wars. The 24 close-up shots of soldiers disfigured in battle in a section titled "The Visage of the War" are perhaps the most disturbing (see Figure 6.4). As Sander Gilman explains,

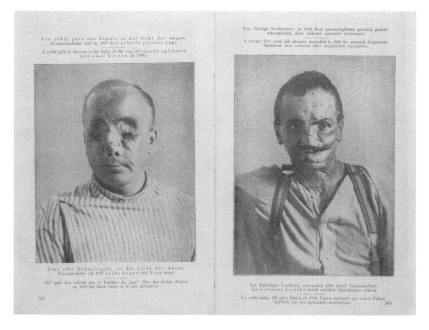

Figure 6.4 From Ernst Friedrich's *Krieg dem Kriege! War Against War! Guerre à la Guerre! Oorlog An Den Oorlog!* (1924)

"whole bodies and all parts of bodies were being shattered in the war, but the facial wounds were often the worst, because in the trenches the face was the most exposed part of the body, as the soldiers peeped over the embankments at the enemy" (1999, 157). The book was "denounced by the government and by veterans' and other patriotic organizations— in some cities the police raided bookstores, and lawsuits were brought against the public display of the photographs" (Sontag 2003, 15). The Berlin Police removed them from the shopwindow of the Anti-War Museum on 30 September 1924 and further display was prohibited.

Carol Poore has identified part of the problem: "With the 2.7 million disabled or permanently ill veterans who returned from the battlefield of World War I, disability came into view in the public sphere in Germany in a different way and to a greater extent than ever before" (2007, 7). While the majority of seriously wounded soldiers used to die from infections or other complications, "by World War I, however, medical advances enabled many more soldiers to survive previously mortal wounds" (Poore 2007, 25). In 1916—in the middle of the war—when the number of war-disabled was still relatively low, one commentator, referring to facial injuries, wrote: "The special characteristic of this type of invalidism . . . is loss in an aesthetic sense, that is, inferiority in outward appearance" (quoted in Poore 2007, 25). Although surgeons attempted a host of new procedures with the means of the time, such as skin grafts, nose and chin reconstructions, and fixing gaping holes in soldiers' faces, they were only partly successful. The physical aspect of disabled, amputated, and disfigured soldiers was judged offensive and raised controversies over whether or not they should be seen in public. As reported by Poore, "journalists often criticized these veterans from an aesthetic standpoint for offensively confronting the postwar public. On 26 November, 1919, for example, the newspaper *Deutsche Tageszeitung* took men to task 'who . . . present an ugly sight in the streets and squares of the big cities'" (2007, 16). While the reality seemed harsh to deal with, artists could somehow manage to transfigure the cripple. Referring to Dix's 50 *War* engravings, the newspaper *Süddeutsche Zeitung* wrote in 1924 that "the substance of these apparitions would be unendurable if a great creative capacity had not subjected the horror to the forms of art" (Löffler 1982, 69). The same can be said about Grosz and Beckmann but not *War against War!*

All these images contrast highly with the idealization of healthy and athletic bodies in the 1920s, when physical education and body culture were actively encouraged by public health services and through the media and health fairs, giving rise to a cult of the body. According to Anton Kaes, "the emphasis on the strong masculine body also compensated for the war-torn bodies on display in the streets of the republic" (2009, 140). One of the most influential books, *Der Mensch und die Sonne* by Hans Surén—a former army physical training officer—came out in 1924 and was translated into English in 1927 (see Figure 6.5). He argued that

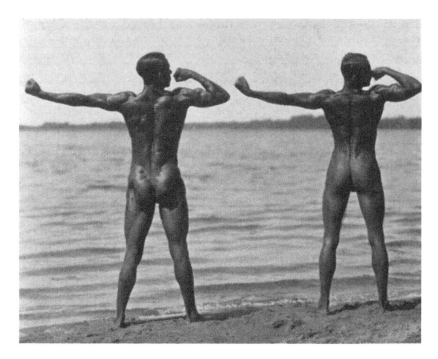

Figure 6.5 From Hans Surén's *Man and Sunlight* (1927)

his "new conception of gymnastics, sport and training" (1927, x) would "restore health and strength to the race" at a time when "around us lurk decline, disease, and death" (179). He praised "the power of health and beauty in [a] trained body" (viii), achieved through "gymnastics—air, and sunlight," where it was "necessary to be naked" (x). While in Surén's view "such bodies . . . give the assurance of future betterment" (viii), the "new paths" (x) he took in his "quest for the perfection of the whole body" (176) were nonetheless deeply rooted in the past, for he argued that "nakedness and gymnastics were, centuries ago, the basis of the health and strength of the Greek race" (122) and that "the Olympic spirit" and "the age of Olympus," as symbols of "this culture of physical and mental health . . . gave eternal models and examples to aftertime" (176–179). To him, "placed in . . . nature, the [naked] human body finds its most ideal manifestation" (7). Consequently, his book is full of photos, mostly of men, nude or in athletic slips, women, and children taking part in various gymnastic exercises and poses outdoors, either individually or in group.

Even if the cult of the body and nakedness reached a peak in popularity during the Weimar Republic, it was not new to Germany. As early as 1893, Heinrich Pudor had published *Naked People* and, in 1906, "Nudity in Art and Life," which praised "the ideal beauty of the ancient

Greeks" and argued that "so-called nudity was natural" for the Greeks (1992, 109, 111). Richard Ungewitter had written several books on nudism since 1903, dealing with a range of issues from art and culture to morality; all contained nude photos. And so did journals, like *Die Schönheit*, which in 1907 "won a case in the federal courts to be permitted to print photos of nude men and women as photography was considered a modern art form" (Krüger 199, 137). Ungewitter also was prosecuted for distribution of obscene material, but all legal procedures failed by 1913. While another book, *Den Freien die Welt* by Walther Brauns, published the same year as *Der Mensch und die Sonne*, contained full frontal nude photos of both women and men, Surén nonetheless felt he had to deal with the erotic potential of the nude to prevent his "pure motives" from being "misunderstood and maligned" and to avoid accusation of immorality; he insisted that "the pictures illustrating this book show men as embodiments of health and strength" (1927, viii) and their bodies "give a higher expression to purity and beauty" (126). He made a clear distinction between "natural nakedness in the midst of sunlight and nature" and the obscene nakedness in "our morally debased civilisation . . . the degrading naked dances in cabarets and saloons," which "mostly has the effect of mere exposure and therefore coarseness" (70). To be "transfigured by godlike purity" (7), bodies had to appear as "magnificent bronzed figures, their skins tended, oiled and divested of superfluous hair" (180).

Although Surén affirms that "it is the sacred duty of everyone to help, by active individual hygiene, in the great work for the benefit of the race and of humanity," his gymnastics, "fundamental views and doctrines" (1927, x), were clearly addressed to the youth. Like Pudor and Ungewitter, he associated trained bodies with art because their "strength and beauty . . . inspire the artist" (135); a sun-tanned, "brown body [is] like a statue in bronze" (146); and "trained naked bodies to be models . . . must give the impression of statues" (180). "Ideal manifestations" of the body, he writes, can be seen in "the magnificent figures which ancient Greece immortalised in marble" (176). While Surén fails to consider the links gymnastics and games had with warfare in ancient Greece, and even if he is critical of German military training (179, 183), his preface mentions issues of "national existence" and "national decline" (viii), the importance of "patriotism" (ix) and "racial upbuilding" (x). As pointed out by Kaes, "Surén's emphasis on the patriotic dimensions of gymnastics had itself a long history, dating back to Friedrich Ludwig Jahn's belief in the early nineteenth century that only well-trained bodies would be capable of defending the nation" (2009, 140). The defeat of Prussia by Napoleonic troops in 1806 had prompted Jahn to launch a program of outdoor physical exercise that he believed would restore the spirits of his countrymen by developing their physical and moral strengths, with the objective of fighting off the invader from the German states.

Wege zu Kraft und Schönheit, subtitled in its English version *A Film about Modern Body Culture*, released in 1925, was the first full-length film dedicated exclusively to body culture. It capitalized on the widespread interest in athletics and physical culture to become one of the most popular films of that period. Just like Surén and life reformers, Prager and Kaufmann emphasize the contrast between ancient Greece and present-day Germany, presumed to be morally and physically degenerating, to support modern physical culture and an open-air active lifestyle. While the film deplores the damaging effects of modern city life and factory work on people, it praises the ancient cult of sports and body worship as if they were the embodiment of a lost ideal to be recovered in the present day. In one sequence, for example, city-life and night-life are contrasted with a historic flashback that reconstructs athletic outdoor activities at a Greek gymnasium, from sprinting and discus throwing to wrestling and boxing. In showing athletes performing more or less naked and women in a Roman public bathhouse, the film suggests that people should imitate the ancients in their everyday life. The film also systematically refers to Greek art. It opens with three successive full-screen shots: a Greek temple, a statue of *Artemis with a Doe*, and *Apollo Belvedere*. In a later scene, a female nude statue—a clear reference to the *Capitoline Aphrodite*—comes to life in front of museum visitors (see Figure 6.6). Compared to the physical appearance of the visitors, Britta Herdegen suggests that "the nude Venus appears as the epitome of physical beauty, health, and harmony, providing a role model for spectators to emulate and thereby reform their destructive lifestyles" (2012, 156). Later in the film, the staging of the *Judgment of Paris* recalls one of Rubens' painting of the myth (see Figure 6.7). While the film "strikes today's eye as an unintentionally comic melange," Theodore Rippey reminds us that "Weimar-era critics, however, took this film as an impressive and important part of an emerging body culture" (2010, 182). Michael Hau has shown that by the turn of the twentieth century, "for life reformers and for some regular physicians, physical beauty was an indicator of a healthy constitution. . . . This holism was tied to aesthetic assumptions—for instance, that a healthy and beautiful body was characterized by the harmonious and purposeful interaction of its constituent parts. Such assumptions were similar to the aesthetic assumptions . . . both suggested that the human organism could be judged intuitively as a coherent whole (as one would judge a work of art)" (2003, 6). Hence they "offered gender-specific representations of the ideal: statues of Hercules and Apollo embodied the masculine ideals of beauty and strength, and statues of Venus gave form to the feminine ideal" (Hau 2003, 33).

In their admiration of the Greek body, life reformers, physicians, and naturists such as Pudor, Ungewitter, and Surén, echo the words of Winckelmann's influential *Reflections on the Imitation of Greek Works in Painting and Sculpture*, published in 1755. Winckelmann wished to revive

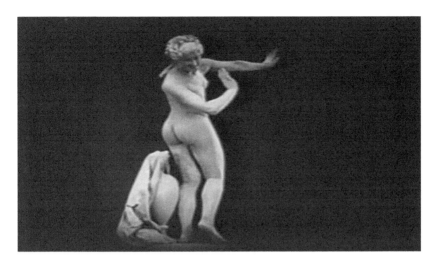

Figure 6.6 Wege zu Kraft und Schönheit [Ways to Strength and Beauty] (1925) screenshot (09:12)

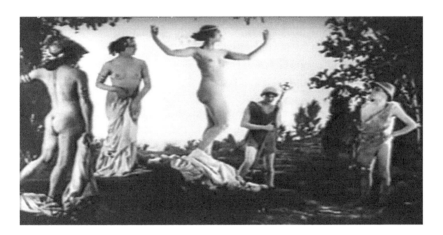

Figure 6.7 Wege zu Kraft und Schönheit [Ways to Strength and Beauty] (1925) screenshot (18:02)

classical Greek art and ideals and contrasted the greatness of ancient Greek artists with what he perceived as the inferiority of the artists of his own time, who, he thought, could not create great artworks because there were no living models that had the physical beauty of ancient Greeks. Their bodies were so beautiful, he argued, because they practiced "physical exercises . . . and trained from infancy in wrestling and swimming" (1987, 7); their art was great because "the schools for artists were the gymnasia, where young people . . . performed their physical exercises in the nude" (11) and exercise gave their bodies "strong and manly contours which the masters then imparted to their statues" (7). *Wege zu Kraft und Schönheit* is reinforced by texts with similar arguments: the film opens with a quote praising Greek antiquity attributed to Goethe, followed by statements that owe to Winckelmann and Nietzsche, such as: "harmonious proportions of the body was the ideal of the ancient Greeks"; "it is not enough to study the works of the ancient Greeks and admire them"; and "we ourselves must strive to emulate the ancient Greeks." Later, Goethe is cited again: "It is when we look back to antiquity, that we for the first time seem to be in a position to understand ourselves and grasp the possibilities of mankind"; and Schiller: "Grace is beauty of movement." Interestingly enough, these two became leaders of the movement known as German Classicism in the late eighteenth century, after having been influenced by Winckelmann. As Jason Geary observes, "for Goethe, ancient Greece had come to represent an ideal that held the promise of stimulating a German cultural and artistic rebirth" (2014, 17). Schiller believed Greek antiquity had been the period in the history of humanity when the individual lived in total unity and harmony with oneself and with nature, but this was destroyed by modern civilization and industrialization. By the late nineteenth century, as Kaes reminds us, "Nietzsche's glorification of the heroic body as an antidote to decadence and degeneration . . . was also widely known" (2009, 140). *Wege zu Kraft und Schönheit* refers to German thinkers not only to endorse gymnastics, sports, dance, and an open-air active lifestyle but to establish very strong ties between Germans and antiquity.

Film critic Siegfried Kracauer alleged that "all these documentaries excelled in evasiveness" as "they mirrored the beautiful world," not "real-life incidents" (1947, 143). *Wege zu Kraft und Schönheit* is no exception to him as it "diverted contemporaries from the evils of the time which no calisthenics would remedy" (143), evils such as postwar social and political unrest, inflation, and soaring unemployment. Rippey discusses how the film denounces the damaging effects of industrialization and mechanization on people, thereby "identifying the body as the prime recipient of the damage of economy and society" and proposing "corporal optimization as the prime means of undoing that damage" (2010, 195). However, he finds that "exercise or working [out] . . . does little to alter those conditions" (195), and notes that "at no point, does the film hint that the timeless model is itself rife with ideology and sociological contingency" (194). It seems as if the film directors were blinded by visions of a world of physical and natural beauty. As with Surén's book, the boundaries between ascetic nakedness and eroticism are unclear. Herdegen argues that the film managed to avoid censorship "through deliberately artistic representations of the nude body that link ancient traditions of physical culture with modern preoccupation with health and fitness" and "by incorporating elements of high-art forms that enjoyed the stamp of legitimacy. The film thus made public nudity acceptable by tying it to Greco-Roman tradition" (2012, 154, 155). The last aspect about *Wege zu Kraft und Schönheit* to be considered here concerns the military training, drills, and parades at the end of the film, which are highlighted with texts declaring that "physical training" is practiced "in many countries only during military service" and that "today sports, not military drills, are the source of a nation's strength." Such statements need to be interpreted in light of the postwar context in which defeated Germany was not allowed to have military service and was excluded from the Olympic Games of 1920 and 1924. To compensate for what was lost, the Germans would presumably have shifted their sense of nationhood and power to exercise and sport. As we have seen with Jahn, the connections between body culture and preparedness for war are deeply rooted in the rise of nationalism in the early 1800s. The motives for promoting sport and exercise were the same in every country: to improve the health of populations, have fit workers for industrial production and ensure military readiness of youth.

Using similar strategies centered on youth, sports, and the cult of the body, *Olympia* documented and glorified the 1936 Olympic Games in Berlin. This two-part film written, directed, and produced by Riefenstahl under the Nazis, was acclaimed internationally when released in 1938 and won several prestigious awards at film festivals in Europe and Japan. Part One, "Festival of the Nations," opens on visual metaphors that evoke the origins of the Olympics through architectural ruins and associate the ideal and godlike beauty to Greek sculpture and bodies of athletes in Greek antiquity. The lyrical prologue, lasting around 20 minutes, is best described by Riefenstahl:

> In my mind's eye, I could see the ancient ruins of the classical Olympic sites slowly emerging from the paths of fog and the Greek temples and sculptures drifting by: Achilles and Aphrodite, Medusa and Zeus, and then the discus thrower of Myron. I dreamed that this statue changed into a man of flesh and blood, gradually starting to swing the discus in slow motion. The sculptures turned into Greek temple dancers dissolving in flames, the Olympic fire igniting the torches to be carried from the temple of Zeus to modern Berlin of 1936—a bridge from Antiquity to the present.
>
> (1993, 171)

The rest of "Festival of the Nations" covers the final competitions and the medal ceremonies in various individual track and field sports, such as throwing, jumping, and running, and the men and women relays. Part Two, "Festival of Beauty," begins with poetic views of nature in harmony with mankind: men run along a watercourse at daybreak, then wash and birch in a sauna, dive and swim naked. This sequence calls to mind a passage from *Der Mensch und die Sonne* where Surén writes: "When early morning borders the distant summer cloudlets with gold, and larks exult over the field and meadow . . . rove and run in free and wealthy nakedness" (1927, 59). After the prologue, the film goes on to show athletes warming up and training, more final competitions in individual sports, team sports, and, lastly, the swimming and diving events. The film ends on the Olympic flame extinguishing. Parallels are easily drawn between *Olympia* and *Wege zu Kraft und Schönheit*, shot 11 years earlier and in which Riefenstahl had featured: both films hail gymnastics and sports, and look back to Greek civilization, temples, and sculptures to showcase athletic bodies as well as fictional reenactments of ancient athletic activities. One of *Olympia*'s most famous and written about segments, in which the *Discobolus* metamorphoses into a modern athlete (the 1935 decathlon champion Erwin Huber) (see Figure 6.8), recalls the statue of Aphrodite coming to life in *Wege zu Kraft und Schönheit*.

Riefenstahl's shots of Zeus, the Olympics originating as a religious festival in his honor, and Aphrodite, the goddess of beauty, are justified. Those of Achilles, a legendary hero in the Trojan War, and Medusa, who had the power of turning into stone anyone who looked into her eyes, are odd. The statue of a reclining muscular nude man, apparently asleep, is intriguing (see Figure 6.9). Details not clearly visible in the film, such as the wreath of ivy on his shaggy hair, the panther skin on which he lies down, and his tail are the attributes of a Greek satyr or Roman faun. This

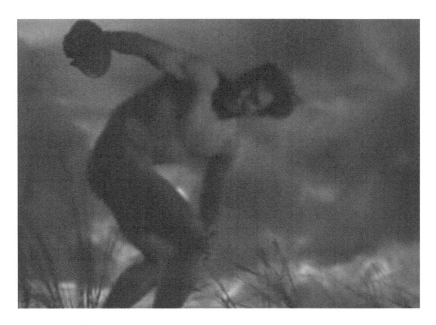

Figure 6.8 Olympia. Part 1 (1938) screenshot (07:08)

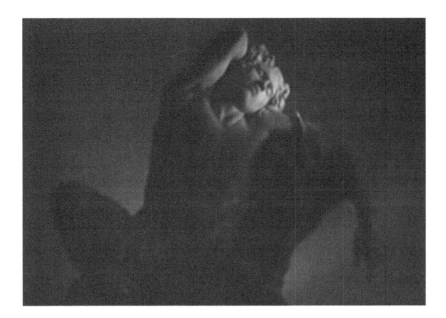

Figure 6.9 Olympia. Part 1 (1938) screenshot (05:52)

sculpture is commonly known as the *Sleeping Satyr* or *Barberini Faun.* While it may meet some standard of beauty, this mythological creature is part-human, part-animal, half-civilized, half-wild, and represents the barbaric side of human nature and does not fit with the ideals of health and sports championed in the film or by the Olympic Games. As followers of the god of wine Dionysus, or Bacchus, these creatures were known for drinking, dancing, chasing the nymphs, and for their riotous living and orgiastic behavior. Could the *Barberini Faun* be sleeping off a bacchanal? He strikes as the opposite of other statues in *Olympia.* In light of James Pitsula's critical comparative analysis of the 1936 Olympics, the presence of a satyr brings a new interpretation to the film. Pitsula shows how the principles of modern Olympism support the erroneous "view that the classical Games fostered peace in the same way that the modern Olympics are supposed to do" and are "a model of international amenity and brotherly cooperation" (2004, 13). For him, "the confusion can be traced to Pierre de Coubertin, the founder of the modern Games, who idealized the Greeks and made them out to be paragons of the harmonious development of mind, body, and spirit" (2).

Much of Pitsula's interpretation of the ancient Olympics rests on the writings of Nietzsche, "whose interpretation of Greek culture diverged markedly from that of the German Classicists who followed Winckelmann's lead" (2004, 7). For Nietzsche, writes Pitsula, "the driving force behind Hellenic culture was not reason leading to harmonious development

(Winckelmann's 'noble simplicity and quiet grandeur') but, rather, 'contest, the striving to surpass and overcome'" (8). Nietzsche saw that "the ancient Greeks had a darker, primitive side. They were not 'humane' and 'civilized' in the modern sense of those terms" (Pitsula 2004, 2): Nietzsche associated this aspect of Greek culture with Dionysus, "the god of chaos and destruction, fertility and productivity, joyful intoxication and abandonment [who represents] 'the most primitive and archaic spirit of Greek history,' as well 'the realm of primitive instincts and urges,'" as Pitsula puts it (8). He opposed Dionysus to Apollo, the god of light, music, and harmony, who stands for the Classicist view of ancient Greek culture—Winckelmann, Goethe, and Schiller, among others. In Rose Pfeffer's words, Nietzsche contends that "[t]he Dionysian elements of barbarism and titanism were as fundamental in Greek culture as were Apollonian elements of sublimity and measure" (1972, 37). It is the union of Apollo and Dionysus, in Nietzsche's view, that made possible the genius and accomplishments of Greek culture. However brief his apparition may be in Riefenstahl's film, the satyr, a follower of Dionysus, challenges the modern values associated with the Olympic Games and could be interpreted in line with the original spirit of the games—the reference to Achilles also. John Hoberman affirms that in the age of fascism, there was "an ideological compatibility between the IOC [International Olympic Committee] elite and the Nazis based on a shared ideal of aristocratic manhood and the value system that derived from their glorification of the physically perfect male as the ideal human being" (1995, 17).

Pitsula also observes that "in the militaristic culture of ancient Greece, it was not always easy to separate the rhetoric of sport from that of war" (2004, 16). As Finley and Pleket remark, "athletes continued to be praised . . . comparisons continued to be drawn between athletics and war, and in the glory to be gained by both" (1976, 21–22). It is clear from Homer's *Iliad* and from other ancient texts that "at that time athletics were a normal diversion of the warrior class" (Harris 1964, 48). The 1936 Games and the film *Olympia* indeed give a picture different from the previous Games. Many have commented on the way in which Riefenstahl captured "the militaristic nature of the organization, particularly the opening ceremony" (Hart-Davis 1971, 242), during which she filmed the "Parade of Nations," where athletes from one country after another march into the stadium and German athletes in military uniform give Hitler the Nazi salute. Germans in military uniforms appear throughout the film, be it Olympic officials, cavalry officers competing in the equestrian events, or athletes—captains and lieutenants—receiving their medals (see Figure 6.10). The outcome of the Berlin Games made obvious the new stakes of body culture: having won a total of 89 medals—of which 33 were gold—Germany emerged victorious from the competitions, clearly superior to other competing nations and way ahead of the US in second rank with 56 medals. Until then, exercise had been regarded

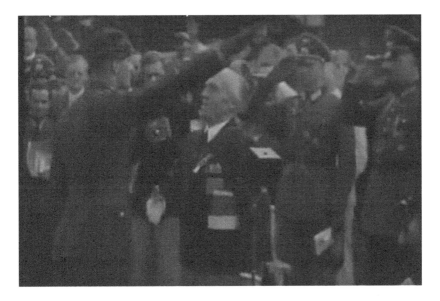

Figure 6.10 Olympia. Part 2 (1938) screenshot (31:35)

as a matter of public health and preparation for war. Now, international sport competition was seen in terms of national prestige and racial superiority. In the opinion of Kaes, Riefenstahl had managed to "perfect the analogy between the athlete's body and the national body. . . . Body culture, in short, had become a realm in which patriotism could be openly displayed" (2009, 140). Furthermore, as Pitsula recounts, "immediately prior to the opening ceremonies, Hitler visited the Langemarck memorial Hall, where he paid tribute to German youth who had sacrificed their lives during the First World War. By this action he symbolically merged the struggles of soldiers on the field of battle with those of the athletes on the field of sport" (2004, 17). With its shifts from documentary truth to fiction about the Games, *Olympia* suggests correlations between athletics, beauty, classical art, ancient Greece and military strength, much more than *Wege zu Kraft und Schönheit* and *Der Mensch und die Sonne* did, while they all avoid to address the consequences of First World War on the soldiers' bodies.

Hitler, who had established a harsh dictatorship by the mid-1930s, did not hesitate to contrast the "new human type" (Hitler 1992, 230) with the maimed, deformed, and disabled. Using the rhetoric of war, he launched a "cultural cleansing" (228) in complement to his racist and eugenic policies. To make his point very clear, two major exhibitions were held in Munich in 1937: the Great German Art Exhibition—a showcase for official art and the first of eight annual exhibitions—and *Degenerate Art*, which included over 600 works by 112 modern artists, mostly Germans. In his inaugural speech at the Great German Art Exhibition on 18 July 1937, Hitler attacked modern art—Impressionism, Cubism, Futurism, and Dadaism—for not being genuine, eternal, and German. In his view, "pseudo-artists" fabricated "deformed cripples and cretins, women who inspire only disgust, men who are more like wild beasts, children who, if they were alive, would be regarded as God's curse" (230). He asserted that "tremendous efforts are being made . . . to make our men, boys, lads, girls, and women more healthy and thereby stronger and more beautiful" (230). For him, "the function of art can only be to symbolize the vitality of this development" of the people (230). He ended his speech by determining that "many of our young artists will recognize the path they will have to take; they will draw inspiration from the greatness of the time in which we all live" (232). Like Huelsenbeck in his manifesto, Hitler called for art and artists to be a reflection of their time. However, times had radically changed and the Nazi perspective negated the not-so-distant past: Sabine Brantl indicates that "special significance was given, in particular after 1939, to depictions of soldiers and war scenes that clearly fulfilled a propaganda purpose. Soldiers, often portrayed as heroic fighters and in aggressive poses, stood for the ideal of German manhood" (2017, 86). On 10 July 1938, at the second Great German Art Exhibition, Hitler praised the recent acquisition of the *Discobolus* (see Figure 6.11), the classical

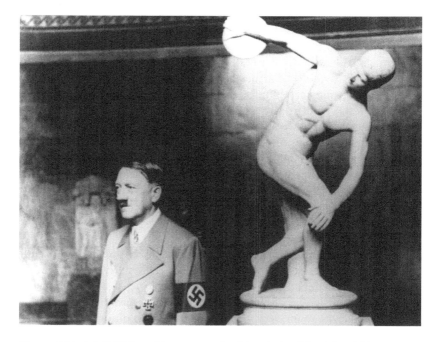

Figure 6.11 Adolf Hitler with a statue of a *Discobolus*, Munich (1938)
Photo © INTERFOTO/Alamy Stock Photo.

statue featured in *Olympia*: "May you all then realize how glorious man already was back then in his corporeal beauty, and that we can speak of progress only if we have attained like perfection or if we manage to surpass this level. . . . And may you all strive for beauty and perfection so that you shall also stand the test of time" (quoted in Domarus 1992, 1127).

Hiltler's programmatic discourse concerned not only art but the physical aspect of Germans. Like Surén and others, he sounds like Winckelmann who had written that "the only way for us to become great . . . is to imitate the ancients" (1987, 5). As he had declared in his speech the previous year: "Never before was humanity in its external appearance and perceptions closer to the ancient world than it is today. This type of human, which we saw last year during the Olympic games . . . is the 'type' of the new age" (1992, 230).

Concerns with degeneration in people, culture, and the arts had already been voiced in the late nineteenth century by Wilhelm Schallmeyer, Max Nordau, and Nietzsche. To illustrate degeneration, Paul Schultze-Naumburg had reproduced modern artworks next to photos of individuals with deformities and diseases in *Kunst und Rasse*, published in 1928, which, unsurprisingly, was reedited in 1938. The Nazi ideology of purification resulted in the elimination of millions of "undesirable" bodies in concentration and extermination camps. Everything progressive or critical stood as a threat and had to be eliminated by force. The Brown Shirts regularly smashed the windows of the Anti-War Museum and tore pictures and documents from its walls. Friedrich was charged with high treason and left Germany in December 1933. Works of art deemed degenerate were confiscated from art institutions and private owners. Some 17,000 works were acquired in this way. The majority were sold on the international art market; the remaining "1004 oil paintings and sculptures as well as 3825 drawings, watercolours and graphic illustrations were burnt as part of a 'fire drill'" (Brantl 2017, 96), in the courtyard of the main fire station in Berlin on 20 March 1939. While gymnastics and exercises had originally been driven by nationalistic motivations and a will to develop physical and moral strength, by the turn of the twentieth century equations were made between health, athletics, beauty, and classical art, as if Greek statues were realistic representations and not idealized bodies. As Karl Toepfer says so well, "Of course, we know that healthy bodies are not necessarily beautiful, and beautiful bodies are not necessarily healthy; healthy bodies are not necessarily strong, nor are strong bodies necessarily healthy; bodies are not necessarily beautiful because they are strong, and strong bodies are only occasionally beautiful" (1997, 33). Beauty is but a subjective, normative, and changing concept. Whether for the sake of art, work productivity or warfare, the body was either intrumentalized or—to use Foucault's term—disciplined between the two World Wars in Germany. No matter the ideals it proposed, the cult of the body did little to free the individual from or compensate for the ills of war.

References

Brantl, Sabine. 2017. *Haus der Kunst, Munich: A Locality and Its History in National Socialism*. Munich: Allitera Verlag.

Carden-Coyne, Ana. 2009. *Reconstructing the Body: Classicism, Modernism, and the First World War*. Oxford: Oxford University Press.

Domarus, Max. 1992. *Hitler: Speeches and Proclamations 1932–1945*. Vol. 2. Translated by Chris Wilcox and Mary Fran Gilbert. Wauconda, IL: Bolchazy-Carducci Publishers.

Eberle, Matthias. 1985. *World War I and the Weimar Artists: Dix, Grosz, Beckmann, Schlemmer*. Translated by John Gabriel. New Haven: Yale University Press.

Finley, Moses, and Henri Willy Pleket. 1976. *The Olympic Games: The First Thousand Years*. Toronto: Clarke, Irwin & Co.

Friedrich, Ernst. 1924. *Krieg dem Kriege! War against War! Guerre à la Guerre! Oorlog an Den Oorlog!* Berlin: Freie Jugend.

Geary, Jason. 2014. *The Politics of Appropriation: German Romantic Music and the Ancient Greek Legacy*. Oxford: Oxford University Press.

Gilman, Sander L. 1999. *Making the Body Beautiful: A Cultural History of Aesthetic Surgery*. Princeton: Princeton University Press.

Grosz, George. 1946. *A Little Yes and a Big No: The Autobiography of George Grosz*. Translated by Lola Sachs Dorin. New York: Dial Press.

Harris, Harold Arthur. 1964. *Greek Athletes and Athletics*. London: Hutchinson.

Hart-Davis, Duff. 1971. *Hitler's Games: The 1936 Olympics*. New York: Harper & Row.

Hau, Michael. 2003. *The Cult of Health and Beauty in Germany*. Chicago, IL: University of Chicago Press.

Herdegen, Britta. 2012. "16 March 1925: *Wege zu Kraft und Schönheit* Educates Audiences in the Art of Nudity." In *A New History of German Cinema*, edited by Jennifer M. Kapczynski and Michael D. Richardson, 153–159. Rochester: Camden House.

Hitler, Adolf. 1992. "Speech Dedicating the House of German Art." Translated by Dieter Kuntz. In *Inside Hitler's Germany: A Documentary History of Life in the Third Reich*, edited by Benjamin Sax and Dieter Kuntz, 225–232. Lexington, MA: D.C. Heath & Company.

Hoberman, John. 1995. "Toward a Theory of Olympic Internationalism." *Journal of Sport History*, 22 (1): 1–37.

Huelsenbeck, Richard. 1993. "Dada Manifesto." In *German Expressionism, Documents from the End of the Wilhelmine Empire to the Rise of National Socialism*, edited by Rose-Carol Washton Long, 266–269. New York: Macmillan.

Kaes, Anton. 2009. *Shell Shock Cinema: Weimar Culture and the Wounds of War*. Princeton, NJ: Princeton University Press.

Kracauer, Siegfried. 1947. *From Caligari to Hitler: A Psychological History of the German Film*. Princeton, NJ: Princeton University Press.

Löffler, Fritz, and Otto Dix. 1982. *Otto Dix, Life and Work*. New York: Holmes & Meier.

Long, Rose-Carol Washton, ed. 1993. *German Expressionism, Documents from the End of the Wilhelmine Empire to the Rise of National Socialism*. New York: Macmillan.

Murray, Ann. 2012. "Reformed Masculinity: Trauma, Soldierhood and Society in Otto Dix's War Cripples and Prague Street." *Artefact: Journal of the Irish Association of Art Historians* 6: 16–31.

Pfeffer, Rose. 1972. *Nietzsche: Disciple of Dionysus.* Lewisburg: Bucknell University Press.

Pitsula, James M. 2004. "The Nazi Olympics: A Reinterpretation." *Olympika: The International Journal of Olympic Studies* 13: 1–26.

Poore, Carol. 2007. *Disability in Twentieth-Century German Culture.* Ann Arbor: The University of Michigan Press.

Pudor, Heinrich. 1992. "Nudity in Art and Life (1906)." *Journal of Homosexuality* 22 (1–2): 109–114.

Reily, Lucia, Helena Panhan, and Ariane Tupinambá. 2009. "Early Evidence of Low-Tech Communication in an Otto Dix Painting of 1920." *Augmentative and Alternative Communication* 25 (4), December: 217–224.

Riefenstahl, Leni. 1993. *Leni Riefenstahl: A Memoir.* New York: St. Martin's Press.

Rippey, Theodore F. 2010. "The Body in Time: Wilhelm Prager's *Wege zu Kraft und Schönheit* (1925)." In *The Many Faces of Weimar Cinema*, edited by Christian Rogowski, 182–197. Rochester: Camden House.

Schmidt, Paul F. 1993. "Max Beckman's *Hell*." In *German Expressionism, Documents from the End of the Wilhelmine Empire to the Rise of National Socialism*, edited by Rose-Carol Washton Long, 151–153. New York: Macmillan.

Sontag, Susan. 2003. *Regarding the Pain of Others.* New York: Picador.

Surén, Hans. 1927. *Man and Sunlight.* Translated from the German 67th edition by David Arthur Jones. Slough: Sollux.

Toepfer, Karl. 1997. *Empire of Ecstasy: Nudity and Movement in German Body Culture, 1910–1935.* Berkeley: University of California Press.

Winckelmann, Johann Joachim. 1987. *Reflections on the Imitation of Greek Works in Painting and Sculpture 1755.* Translated by Elfriede Heyer and Roger C. Norton. La Salle, IL: Open Court.

7   Representing AIDS

KS Lesions, US Visual Culture, and the Body as Canvas (1983–1993)

Kylo-Patrick R. Hart

By the late 1970s in the United States, medical professionals had identified a growing number of young men living in the urban areas of Los Angeles, Miami, New York, and San Francisco who were suffering from a rare form of skin cancer, Kaposi's sarcoma (KS), which has "a striking visual presentation, bluish or purple-brown nodules that appear on the skin" (Gilman 1988, 246). What particularly stood out to them is that, while this dermatological condition in the past had rarely been fatal, many of these young men were now dying within several months of being diagnosed with it, often in conjunction with *Pneumocystis carinii* pneumonia (PCP; Gilman 1988; Hart 2000).

By 1981, it was further noted that a common attribute among many of these men was that they engaged regularly in homosexual sexual activities, which led physicians initially to refer to the resulting KS/PCP condition as GRID, which stood for gay-related immune deficiency (Gilman 1988; Hart 2000). Accordingly, by the time the US Centers for Disease Control (CDC) changed the label for this condition to AIDS (which stands for acquired immune deficiency syndrome) in the fall of 1982, it had already been socially constructed as a "gay cancer" or "gay plague" in the minds of many Americans (Hart 2000). This is the case even though, as early as August 1981, women and other heterosexual patients with AIDS had been reported to the CDC (Padgug and Oppenheimer 1992).

When intravenous drug users were added to the list of individuals commonly infected with AIDS, this initial social construction was broadened to include a second type of so-called "guilty" and/or "deviant" group of individuals who were culturally regarded as having contracted AIDS "through their intentional pursuit of 'deviant' and 'immoral' behaviors" (Hart 2000, 39). Such perceptions continued to persist during the pandemic's early years, even after researchers successfully isolated the virus that leads to AIDS in 1983 and labeled it HIV (which stands for human immunodeficiency virus).

It was in that same year, 1983, that popular media and related forms of visual culture in the United States "discovered" AIDS and began to represent it with increasing regularity (Grover 1992). The range of media forms regularly featuring images of people with AIDS during the decade of the 1980s and beyond included art installations, documentaries, films, magazines, newscasts, newspapers, paintings, photographs, posters, television programs, and videos, which together raised important questions about the most appropriate ways to do so (Griffin 2000). The clear majority of images in these various media outlets during the pandemic's early years took their lead from the visual icons of the medical field and its emphasis on prominently featuring KS lesions—the distinctive purple blotches that can often be found covering the faces and bodies of infected individuals—in relation to people with AIDS (Grover 1992).

"As with any other type of visual media content, media professionals readily developed conventions for depicting people in the advanced stages of AIDS—with a primary emphasis on emaciated individuals covered with a substantial number of the purple KS blotches—as a shorthand way to 'routinize the unexpected' [Cook and Colby 1992, 85] that tended to be unsympathetic and reinforced harmful social perceptions of otherness and deviancy in relation to people with AIDS" (Hart 2007, 141). It soon became quite common for individuals who worked with these media forms to seek out the most disfigured and debilitated, visibly ill people with AIDS they could possibly find (Grover 1992). A particularly noteworthy example of this process occurred in the ABC television network's May 1983 *20/20* coverage of AIDS, which passed over numerous male subjects who didn't *look* particularly ill in favor of prominently featuring Kenneth Ramsauer, a 28-year-old male whose once-stunning face had become severely disfigured from Kaposi's sarcoma. The resulting imagery discouraged viewer identification with Ramsauer by contrasting his formerly attractive appearance with the physical grotesqueness caused by KS and AIDS (Grover 1992). In addition, it soon became widely evident that "counter-examples to these canonical AIDS victims [were] systematically excluded . . . by photographers because they [did] not look sick enough" (Treichler 1992, 143).

From the earliest years of the crisis, various concerns were raised in relation to the reception of images of people with AIDS. Some cautioned about how such representations appear to be natural as a result of their continual use and repetition, with the human body serving as both a costume and a canvas for the visual manifestation of AIDS (Kalin 1992, 120, 123). Others emphasized the harm caused when influential visual images strive primarily to emphasize the *difference* of KS-lesion-filled individuals from everyone else in the same society (Grover 1992); in this regard, it is essential to acknowledge that the male homosexuals and IV drug users with prominent KS lesions were implicitly represented as being "polluted" and "cursed" beings (Elbaz and Murbach 1992, 6) or perhaps even "dehumanized monsters" (Kalin 1992, 120). A subset of these concerns pertained to the ongoing circulation of such imagery in society, to the "seemingly independent life of the images" as works of art and the ways they may reappear throughout history, to reinforce outdated cultural perceptions of the pandemic's realities (Gilman 1988, 246). In these important regards, as Sander Gilman has noted, "To explore the semiotics of the disease means to understand not only the overt level of meaning but also the complex confusions that permeate the images of the AIDS patient" (1988, 246).

The immediate goal appears to have been to determine a shorthand way for visually separating "sick" vs. "healthy" individuals in the AIDS crisis (Griffin 2000); the reality that the resulting representational strategies ended up causing antipathy toward certain kinds of people with AIDS was an unfortunate and deleterious consequence (Padgug and Oppenheimer 1992). Jan Zita Grover (1992) has demonstrated the interrelation among how, from the early days of the pandemic, AIDS was represented in the discursive fields of medicine, mainstream and alternative media outlets, and art photography, with a particular emphasis on prominently focusing on KS lesions in order to symbolically create an "us" vs. "them" dichotomy in relation to people with AIDS among members of the so-called "general population." However, the initial goal of this representational approach had much more to do with serving the needs of "conservative morality in a deeply puritanical culture" than with accurately representing the realities of the AIDS crisis and the range of individuals affected by it (Patton 1990, 25). Reinforcing this assessment, Gabriele Griffin has emphasized that "visualization and visibility in the general cultural field, within mainstream, non-specialized (i.e. non-medicalized) contexts, answer to those conventions and idealizations of the representation of the body which conjoin the aesthetic with the moral" (2000, 63).

The growing emphasis on KS lesions in US visual culture corresponded to the shift, in early network news accounts, from describing the initial outbreak of AIDS as "mysterious" and "fascinating" to something that had clearly turned "deadly" and quite threatening (Cook and Colby 1992, 95). In certain regards this is perhaps unsurprising, as epidemics in past centuries often prescribed the "ritual marking of the Other," and KS lesions efficiently served an analogous function in late-twentieth-century visual culture (Elbaz and Murbach 1992, 3). As Mikhaël Elbaz and Ruth Murbach (1992) have demonstrated, history has shown that it is far easier to blame the victims of an epidemic disease whenever they can be conceived of and/or visually represented to be "different." Naturally, several other kinds of images of people with AIDS—including personal snapshots, family portraits, and home videos that did not seek to promote a sense of otherness—were created during the early to mid-1980s in hopes of countering the ones already so common in US visual culture; however, they did not typically receive the same breadth of cultural distribution or display and therefore were far less influential to the social construction of AIDS and people with AIDS in US society (Grover 1992; Hart 2000).

In his writings about the daily realities of personally living with AIDS, film director Derek Jarmin emphasized concerns about the disfigurement caused by Kaposi's sarcoma and how it seemed more horrendous to him than the illness itself, because it publicly marked him as a person with AIDS in the eyes of the entire world (Griffin 2000). With regard to how individuals like Jarmin were regularly represented, Emmanuel Dreuilhe articulated, in his memoir *Mortal Embrace: Living with AIDS*, how "the camera invariably seeks out the 'victims' of the most spectacular battles. Its instinct for the sensational leads it to prefer the bald and wasted AIDS patient with the feverish, [blotchy], haggard look, lying in his hospital bed (preferably with a few tubes up his nose), to his companion who is still able to take care of himself and speak articulately about his condition" (1988, 122).

As such deleterious representational patterns continued, the members of ACT UP, the New York City-based AIDS activist group, began to demand "No more pictures without context" and "Stop looking at us; start listening to us," in their ongoing efforts to communicate that such representations have very real effects on those who are portrayed (Grover 1992, 39–40). Nevertheless, offerings in many media forms frequently remained "frozen" in the visual approaches and narrative strategies established in the earliest years of the 1980s, rather than effectively evolving to reflect the ongoing demographic changes in the AIDS crisis (Watney 1992, 155).

Because media professionals and artists do not create images in a vacuum, it is perhaps to be expected that their resulting representations of AIDS and people with AIDS during the first half of the 1980s were significantly influenced by the ways that physicians and scientific researchers had already been doing so (Grover 1992). However, this sort of default approach to creating and disseminating influential images of the AIDS pandemic, problematic as it was from the onset, became increasingly suspect over time, particularly as that decade continued to unfold. In this regard, Grover raises two important questions about this resulting state of representational affairs: "What does it mean in 1989, when the average life expectancy of a person diagnosed with AIDS is over 20 months, for a photographer to consistently depict PWAs [persons with AIDS] as debilitated, disfigured, *in extremis*? Does it mean the same thing(s) as it did in 1983, when the average life expectancy of a person diagnosed with AIDS was only eight months?" (1992, 24–25). One of the points she makes in her subsequent discussion is that representational approaches that begin at the cultural core (e.g., scientific approaches) tend to turn into "that-which-is-no-longer-debated" as they move to the cultural periphery and become commonplace (Grover 1992, 26).

From the moment the KS-lesion-centered imagery began to surface in US society, members of the gay community "insisted that AIDS must be viewed as a disease and not a divine judgment" and that "persons with AIDS must be seen as human beings with a disease rather than as moral outcasts" (Padgug and Oppenheimer 1992, 259). They further emphasized that people with AIDS have their own voice that must be heard and deserve to be treated with respect at all times (Padgug and Oppenheimer 1992). Nevertheless, as the decade of the 1980s unfolded, while retaining an emphasis on emaciated individuals with visible KS lesions, it became increasingly common for various representations to emphasize the isolation and melancholy of the subjects with AIDS (Gilman 1988). At least in part, from an ideological perspective this was to prevent widespread hysteria by implicitly serving to counter the growing fear that AIDS was a potential danger to everyone, including heterosexuals (Gilman 1988). As Gilman has demonstrated about the resulting representational state of affairs, "The AIDS patient remains the suffering hopeless [gay or drug-injecting] male, both the victim and the source of his own pollution. The AIDS patients are represented iconographically as depressed males, with their sense of their marginality stressed even in those media that are not overtly condemnatory" (1988, 262).

At the time actor Rock Hudson confirmed his AIDS diagnosis in July 1985, it was still quite common for images of people with AIDS in US visual culture to emphasize KS lesions in order to strongly communicate the message that these "marked" individuals were "doomed to die" (Grover 1992, 24). However, Hudson's death just three months later substantially fueled the "heterosexual panic" about HIV/AIDS that vigorously ensued in the popular media, which many regard as a significant "turning point in national consciousness" and eventually resulted in changes to common representational strategies and approaches (Grover 1992, 28–29). Reporting emphases and visual representations pertaining to HIV/AIDS first expanded to emphasize sexually active heterosexuals who are potentially at risk and then to increasingly diverse discourses about women and AIDS (Grover 1992). Such representational shifts make sense at a time when it had become clear that the threat of AIDS in American society "was no longer embodied only in people with visible lesions: it might also be your neighbour (who looked a little effeminate), your boss or secretary. . . . The invisibility of infection threw into question the comfortable categories that had kept anxieties manageable for many 'low-risk' people" (Grover 1992, 35). The resulting collective paranoia stemmed from the growing realization that appearances could be deceiving, as well as from continual exposure to contradictory media images and messages suggesting that a wide range of individuals both *were* and *were not* at risk (Kalin 1992; Watney 1992). Another reason for such shifts was the recognition that AIDS was increasingly becoming a medical condition that individuals live with.

As the decade of the 1980s continued, HIV/AIDS was increasingly culturally regarded as the distinct yet interrelated epidemics of HIV and AIDS (Griffin 2000, 76). In addition, by early 1987 in the United States, "the public understanding of AIDS as a disease not limited to specific marginal groups had begun to grow," and the majority of individuals being tested in New York and San Francisco public AIDS clinics were now heterosexuals (Gilman 1988, 269). This led to a shift, in mainstream media offerings as well as in public health campaigns, toward imagery focusing on individuals with healthy but "at risk" bodies, as opposed to the iconically established iconography of emaciated gay men and IV drug users with prominent KS lesions (Griffin 2000). In addition, during the latter half of the 1980s, "children with AIDS (one percent of total US AIDS cases) received more media attention than the 61 percent of diagnosed cases among gay men" (Grover 1992, 25).

In 1993, *Philadelphia* (directed by Jonathan Demme)—Hollywood's first all-star movie about AIDS starring Tom Hanks and Denzel Washington—premiered, and it ended up luring "hordes of straight viewers to sit through an AIDS movie" addressing the cultural realities of many gay men's lives, often for the first time (Hart 2000, 54). In addition to generating more than $72 million dollars at the box office during the first 18 weeks of its release, this film "brought the theme of AIDS to the attention of a wider general public than any previous film" (Baker 1994, 21). Perhaps unsurprisingly, given audience expectations and the historical era during which it was made, this story of a lawyer, Andrew Beckett (played by Hanks), who gets fired by his firm as a result of his medical condition, focuses quite prominently on KS lesions as its narrative unfolds. For example, it is the appearance of a KS lesion on Beckett's forehead early on that makes his emergent medical condition, which is otherwise unseeable, immediately legible to viewers. It is also a KS lesion noticed by one of the senior partners in Beckett's firm that eventually leads to the suspicion that Beckett may be progressing toward full-blown AIDS (Baker 1994).

However, as *Philadelphia*'s narrative continues and the number of KS lesions on Beckett's body multiplies, these distinctive blotches serve a very different representational function in the film than the similar ones in US visual culture of the decade prior. Upon realizing that his partners have sabotaged him so that they could fire him for professional incompetence after they concluded he is ill, Beckett finds a lawyer and sues. As the corresponding sequences are presented, the film remains sensitive about presenting Beckett's "deteriorating physical condition without morbidly sensationalizing it" (Baker 1994, 23), in contrast to so many of the similar sorts of representations during the decade of the 1980s.

Ultimately and quite significantly, it is the numerous KS lesions in the film that enable Beckett to win his court case. The defense team argues that it would have been difficult for the man's former legal colleagues to see his lesions from a distance, thereby making it impossible for them to know he was a person with AIDS. When the physically fragile Beckett, upon request of the judge, removes his shirt in the courtroom to reveal the numerous prominent lesions on his torso, the blotches evoke significant sympathy among the majority of the surrounding individuals, rather than contempt. In this way, the film "finds in the lesions an efficient way to visibly/physically manifest the topic of difference in relation to illness (here, specifically, HIV/AIDS) and social intolerance toward it. In fact, the moment at which Andy reveals the many KS lesions on his chest in court serves as an updated version of a tableau moment, the point at which, in theatrical melodramas and early silent-film melodramas, all of the characters would freeze in position so that the audience members could more fully comprehend the significance of the moment" (Hart 2000, 143–144). In doing so, it serves significantly to challenge the longstanding "us" vs. "them" dichotomy in US visual culture by reinforcing the virtue of the character of Andrew Beckett and repositioning this KS-lesion-covered gay man as an individual deserving of sympathy at the cultural level, innovatively utilizing the representational conventions of the preceding decade to challenge AIDS discrimination rather than to foster it.

References

Baker, Rob. 1994. *The Art of AIDS: From Stigma to Conscience*. New York: Continuum.

Cook, Timothy E., and David C. Colby. 1992. "The Mass-Mediated Epidemic: The Politics of AIDS on the Nightly Network News." In *AIDS: The Making of a Chronic Disease*, edited by Elizabeth Fee and Daniel M. Fox, 84–122. Berkeley: University of California Press.

Dreuilhe, Emmanuel. 1988. *Mortal Embrace: Living with AIDS*. New York: Hill and Wang.

Elbaz, Mikhaël, and Ruth Murbach. 1992. "Fear of the Other, Condemned and Damned: AIDS, Epidemics and Exclusions." In *A Leap in the Dark: AIDS, Art and Contemporary Cultures*, edited by Allan Klusacek and Ken Morrison, 1–9. Montreal: Véhicule Press.

Gilman, Sander L. 1988. *Disease and Representation: Images of Illness from Madness to AIDS*. Ithaca: Cornell University Press.

Griffin, Gabriele. 2000. *Representations of HIV and AIDS: Visibility Blue/s*. Manchester: Manchester University Press.

Grover, Jan Zita. 1992. "Visible Lesions: Images of the PWA in America." In *Fluid Exchanges: Artists and Critics in the AIDS Crisis*, edited by James Miller, 23–52. Toronto: University of Toronto Press.

Hart, Kylo-Patrick R. 2000. *The AIDS Movie: Representing a Pandemic in Film and Television*. New York: Routledge.

Hart, Kylo-Patrick R. 2007. "Our Bodies, Their Bodies, and (In)Visible Lesions: AIDS, Film Melodramas, and the Transformation from 'Us' versus 'Them' to 'Just Us.'" In *Mediated Deviance and Social Otherness: Interrogating Influential Representations*, edited by Kylo-Patrick R. Hart, 140–152. Newcastle: Cambridge Scholars Publishing.

Kalin, Tom. 1992. "Flesh Histories." In *A Leap in the Dark: AIDS, Art and Contemporary Cultures*, edited by Allan Klusacek and Ken Morrison, 120–135. Montreal: Véhicule Press.

Padgug, Robert A., and Gerald M. Oppenheimer. 1992. "Riding the Tiger: AIDS and the Gay Community." In *AIDS: The Making of a Chronic Disease*, edited by Elizabeth Fee and Daniel M. Fox, 245–278. Berkeley: University of California Press.

Patton, Cindy. 1990. *Inventing AIDS*. New York: Routledge.

Treichler, Paula A. 1992. "Seduced and Terrorized: AIDS and Network Television." In *A Leap in the Dark: AIDS, Art and Contemporary Cultures*, edited by Allan Klusacek and Ken Morrison, 136–151. Montreal: Véhicule Press.

Watney, Simon. 1992. "Short-Term Companions: AIDS as Popular Entertainment." In *A Leap in the Dark: AIDS, Art and Contemporary Cultures*, edited by Allan Klusacek and Ken Morrison, 152–165. Montreal: Véhicule Press.

Part IV
The Punished Body

8 The Criminal's Hair
Forensic Practices (1600–1945)

Willemijn Ruberg

Introduction

Historians generally regard the modern body as an object of discipline. This holds particularly for the criminal's body. Foucault ([1975] 1995) argues that the power of modern criminal justice might not be primarily aimed at the body anymore (since corporal punishment had been abolished) but is now targeted at mind and body in order to discipline people into becoming productive citizens. Whereas Foucault is critical of the modern discourse of Enlightenment as presented by penal reformers, historian Lynn Hunt takes a more positive view on the history of human rights and argued that torture and dishonoring punishments started to disappear in the mid-eighteenth century because of new ideas on the individual ownership of the body, as well as bodily inviolability ([2007] 2008, 30, 141, 234n16). Both aspects seem to be inextricably interwoven in the modern body.

This chapter will explore multiple meanings of the modern body, focusing on the role of hair in penal and forensic practice. At first sight, the notion of discipline seems most applicable here. The few existing histories of hair often refer to discipline by the state or prisons in regard to laws and regulations on haircuts (Pergament 1999) or to the disciplining of (especially) female bodies by practices of hair removal (Herzig 2015). A focus on discipline is certainly relevant when it comes to the criminal's hair, but I would like to propose an additional perspective, taking as a starting point philosopher Gilles Deleuze's notion of the body as something that is always becoming. I am building here on the work of historian Lisa Helps (2007, 128), who proposes to use Deleuze's ideas on the body to conceptualize a new history *through the body* (rather than body history). Helps states that the concept of "embodiment," the specific practices of lived bodies in relation to each other and to cultural discourses, allows us to emphasize not only the effects of systems of power on bodies but also the modes through which bodies *are* in the world (2007, 131–132). For Deleuze, the body is a "social organ whose structure and limits change in relationship with other bodies. It desires to connect to other organic and inorganic bodies to form assemblages" (Helps 2007, 128). This body is at the same time biological, collective, political, and always changing. Deleuze thus emphasizes the body's potential of becoming, asking the (Spinozist) question: "What can a body do?" (Buchanan 1997). Deleuze (1997) gives desire primacy over power and normalization, not denying or rejecting discipline but simply emphasizing the body's potential, which is perhaps closer to Foucault's insight that power is also productive.

This chapter will address the social meanings of hair, starting with those at the forefront of early modern criminal punishment, which seem to disappear with the rise of modern (forensic) science around 1900, when hair becomes disconnected from the body in the new science of criminalistics. But these symbolic meanings reappear briefly after the Second World War, when the hair of numerous girls and women was shaved by emotional groups of people who accused them of having slept with German soldiers. In addition to the role of hair in disciplining practices, I explore the role of hair as an indicator of individual identity in modernity. Modern science has used hair as a means to demarcate the human individual from animals and to underline gender and racial differences, what Joanna Bourke (2011) has called, in short, "what it means to be human." Hair can thus be seen as part of embodiment, as incorporating continually shifting cultural meanings. By growing from the body, but also by taking different shapes according to social and historical context, it might be regarded as an example of the body that is becoming.

Anthropological Theories on Hair

Sociologists and anthropologists have pointed to hair as a powerful symbol of individual and group identity, of gender and sexuality, and also as a mode of self-expression and communication. As sociologist Anthony Synnott states: "Hair not only symbolizes the self but, in a very real sense, it *is* the self since it grows from and is part of the physical human body" (1987, 381). Synnott argues that its power derives from hair being both physical and very personal, and also public. Moreover, because it is malleable, it can indicate shifting identities as well (Synnott 1987, 381). Similarly, anthropologists have researched hair symbolism, particularly focusing on initiation rites, marriage ceremonies, mourning rituals, and the magic attributed to hair by non-Western societies. They show how hair always relates to social rules (Pergament 1999) but can also stand for the total individual, their soul, or their personal power (Leach 1958, 160).

Anthropologist Edmund Leach, in an article on hair published in 1958, agrees with psychoanalyst Charles Berg's interpretation of hair as having a phallic significance (the head being the symbol of the phallus, head hair of semen and hair cutting or shaving seen as symbolic castration). Freud had already underlined hair's fetishistic character, arguing that it is seen as a public, phallic substitute, signifying castration anxiety (Berg

1951). Anthropologist Leach takes an ambivalent position. On the one hand, he agrees with the psychoanalytic focus on sexuality, theorizing that long hair represents unrestrained sexuality, while short hair, tightly bound, or partially shaved hair signifies restricted sexuality and shaved heads symbolize celibacy. On the other hand, Leach finds psychoanalytical theory's emphasis on the universal not valid. Neither does he agree that the libidinal nature of hair rituals was unconscious. Leach states: "In the anthropologist's view, ritually powerful human hair is full of magical potency, not because it is hair but because of the ritual context of its source" (1958, 159).

In an article from 1969, anthropologist Christopher Hallpike criticizes Leach's interpretation. Hallpike makes a plea for an empirical study of symbolism, relating to the world and man's place in it, in contrast to the psychoanalytical emphasis on the workings of the subconscious, which remained theoretical. Hallpike doubts Leach's emphasis on phallicism (the head standing for the phallus, the hair for semen) in ritual as a form of cathartic prophylaxis, to control potentially dangerous emotions. Hallpike moreover counters Leach's argument that shaving and cutting hair equaled castration; instead Hallpike points out that women shave their heads in mourning, so castration could not play a role. Second, Hallpike asks, if head hair symbolized male genitals, what were the meanings of the beard? Third, Hallpike points out that ascetics commonly have long hair. Rather than reducing the use of hair in ritual to symbolic castration, Hallpike proposes another explanation: hair is used in magic to symbolize the person from whom it was taken; since it grows, it is believed to be endowed with vitality (and may be associated with the soul when it comes from the head). Hallpike's main hypothesis is "that long hair is associated with being outside society and that the cutting of hair symbolizes re-entering society, or living under a particular disciplinary regime" (1969, 260). In regard to the latter, he refers to convicts, soldiers, and monks. By contrast, groups with long hair, like intellectuals, juvenile rebels, and women were seen to be less subject to social control. Long hair is, therefore, according to Hallpike, "a symbol of being in some way outside society," which is often associated with animality (1969, 261). In regard to women, following the biblical interpretation, growing long hair is equaled with a separation from society (and a move to religion); shaving hair equals rejoining society; and covering hair equals discipline (women's acceptance of husbands' authority; Hallpike 1969, 263).

These anthropologists thus differ in regard to the symbolism of hair, forwarding hair as symbol of both sexuality and the distance to society, where the proximity to society is interwoven with ideas on gender and the human/animal divide. Anthropologists have furthermore emphasized the symbolics of purity and dirt: Leach (1958, 157) already noted that whereas head hair is often carefully treated, as soon as it is cut off it is seen as dirt or pollution. Similarly, anthropologist Mary Douglas ([1966]

2008) points to the power and danger associated with bodily margins and orifices. Douglas mentions that semen, blood, and excreta were often seen as polluting. Especially feminine margins can be regarded as threatening since they incarnate the permeability of the social body. Douglas and Leach suggest that hair, as an extrusion of the body, becomes dirt due to its structural ambiguity and physical liminality and is therefore in need of control. Hair can thus be seen as a liminal space and a dangerous bodily margin. Ofek (2009) argues that since hair is simply "issuing forth," it traverses the boundary of the body and is perceived as a structural anomaly.

Hair Shaving in the Early Modern Period

Already in Antiquity and the early Middle Ages, the shaving of the head was known as a punishment, mostly for men (Geltner 2014, 62). It is unclear how often hair shaving as punishment was meted out, but several types of law books mention its presence in the early modern Southern and Northern Netherlands. During witch trials in the Netherlands in the seventeenth century, the bodies of several men and women accused of witchcraft were shaved by physicians to search for signs of the devil before they could be tortured (Monballyu 2003, 128–132). In eighteenth-century France, legal manuals also advised both shaving the accused and searching bodily cavities for concealed charms that might protect the accused from the pain of torture. Lisa Silverman (2001, 95) argues that the shaving of the convict's head was part of the ritual of the legal system's shaming and degrading of the accused.

In the early modern period, in several European countries the shaving of criminals' hair (or the burning down or tearing off of the hair) was used as a dishonorable punishment. It was the equivalent of branding, since both made the criminal publicly recognizable and were often used for girls and women accused of adultery or prostitution (de Win 1991, 26, 150; Maes 1947, 423; Virgili 2004, 232). Although hair shaving as punishment seems to have disappeared in modernity, it returns in another shape: for instance, in early twentieth-century Dutch prisons, prisoners were photographed, then their beards were shaved off and their head hair cut short. They experienced this as a loss of identity (Franke 1990, 385–386). It is therefore clear that the meanings of hair in regard to punishment relate to personal identity and honor, gender, sexuality, and humanity.

Nineteenth-Century Science: Hair and Abnormality

In the nineteenth century, several scientists also regarded hair as a sign of identity, character, or insanity. Rebecca Herzig argues that the publication of Darwin's *Descent of Man* in 1871 had a significant impact on, for example, Americans' ideas on body hair. Whereas previously they had explained the presence or absence of hair by referring to divine design or the balance of the humors, now differences in hair type and amount came to be seen as effects of evolution—as the results of competitive selection. Darwin referred to (unconscious) sexual selection to explain the inheritance of disadvantageous bodily characteristics such as the human lack of body hair. However, Darwin's explanation of human hairlessness as a cultivated characteristic (through grooming) seemed difficult to reconcile with the idea of unconscious sexual selection. It therefore remained unclear how the "denudation of man" happened. Although Darwin received much critique, his evolutionary vocabulary influenced later representations of extraordinarily hairy people and other images of hair in which the similarities between man and beast were emphasized. Also, experts became preoccupied with excessive hair, especially in women (Herzig 2015, 55–68). Herzig (2015, 68–71) argues that around 1900, hairiness had been established as a sign of sexual, mental, and criminal deviance.

Late nineteenth-century criminologists and alienists underlined the association between hairiness and mental illness, long hair having long been a sign of lunacy. In the nineteenth century, examining differences in hair became a favored method of medical classification. For instance, in an American lunacy trial in 1851, the lawyer analyzed a hair root sample from the presumed lunatic under the microscope, which he said showed a white, transparent, regularly shaped structure at the end, unlike the dark, distorted, and irregularly shaped structure allegedly "characteristic of insanity" (Herzig 2015, 71–73). Similarly, criminal anthropologists like Cesare Lombroso (1835–1909) also focused on hair when measuring the criminal body. They noted the presence or absence of beards and the prevalence of gray hair or baldness; both were regarded as very rare among criminals, epileptics, and cretins and linked to their "reduced emotional sensibility" (Horn 2003, 14). Lombroso connected the European criminal to the non-European "savage" by referring to many corporeal phenomena, among which thinning hair and curly hair (Horn 2003, 43). Italian physician and criminologist Antonio Marro (1840–1913) stated, "the most bloodthirsty beasts are often hidden behind a hairless and pale face" (Horn 2003, 76). Lombroso and his colleague Guglielmo Ferrero thought that penalties inflicted on vanity, such as the cutting off of the hair or the obligation to wear a certain costume, were appropriate for female criminals (Horn 2003, 141).

This scientific study of hair could also serve to demarcate the races. The Dutch physician Gijsbert A.J. van der Sande (1863–1910) studied hair as part of his anthropometrical research. He labeled eye color, ear shape, and the degree of curliness of the hair. For the latter, he developed a special form (Mak and Bultman 2019). Other anthropologists, like German scholar Rudolf Martin (1864–1925; 1914, 190), designed hair structure schemes for classification in order to provide "objective" measurements. Martin used E. Fischer's "hair color table," a box with fake hair in different colors. Martin (1914, 188–189) designed a chart listing different shapes of hair, from curly to straight. In his textbook, he added instructions on how to examine hair under the microscope but also acknowledged that hairdo, as well as the treatment of hair with water, ointments etc., could change its texture (1914, 190). In this respect, ever-changing hair was different from the skulls and other permanent bodily features of "primitive" people measured by anthropologists.

To summarize, nineteenth and early twentieth-century scientists studied hair to demarcate normal from abnormal individuals. Herzig (2015, 74) argues that around 1920, aversion to body hair had become very strong, influenced by the threat of degeneracy and the associations with atavism, individual pathology, sexual inversion, and mental illness.

Hair and Forensic Science

Scientific developments also influenced the study of the criminal's hair as a means to solving a crime. Before circa 1900, the criminal's hair only functioned as one of the ways to identify criminals and prisoners. Before the advent of identification by photographs (around 1850), a criminal's personal charts also contained a section on "hair" next to bodily features, clothing, etc. In the late nineteenth century, the French police official Alphonse Bertillon designed a system for the measurement of the body of criminals. His anthropometric system included physical descriptions like beard, hair color, and hair growth pattern (Cole 2001, 37).

However, from the mid-nineteenth century, the budding discipline of forensic science showed more interest in hair as a means of identification and, in addition, of tracing evidence. This type of science was stripped of magical connotations and seemingly also of associations with gender, sexuality, or abnormality. The scientific study of hair (trichology) dates from the mid-1800s. Its forensic application started around 1860. The first case of the determination of poison in human hair was published in Johann Ludwig Casper's 1858 textbook on forensic medicine (Sachs 1997, 7). In addition, hairs found on the defendant were compared to the victim's hair in order to establish a link. Forensic hair analysis started to play a major role in courts in the beginning of the 1900s, when criminalistics as an applied science started to blossom. This period witnessed the introduction of fingerprints and now trace evidence was sent to laboratories. In 1901, for example, bloodstains could be accurately attributed to specific species (Watson 2011, 141–143). Thus, the differences between mammals could be pinpointed, contributing to the demarcations between human and animal.

The field of forensic science, focused on trace evidence, expanded rapidly after microscopic hair examination became known in the early twentieth century, although only the species the hair belonged to could be established, without being able to determine its individual, unique aspects (Bisbing 1982). For Hans Gross (1847–1915), the founding father of criminalistics, hair was an important "silent witness," one of the objects found at the crime scene. Hairs found on the hands of a corpse or on clothing could contain the perpetrator's hair; hairs found on a knife or axe could indicate they were from the victim. These hairs needed to be handled meticulously and carefully. The police officer needed to place the hair in marked envelopes and airtight bottles or receptacles. Gross also showed that this type of evidence could help a judge establish the correct identity of the perpetrator (Schreuder 1949, 56, 108).

Gross, whose influential handbook of criminal investigation was first published in 1893, prescribed how to meticulously indicate the position in which the hair was found. He recommended that the hair must be taken with clean hands and placed in a clean bottle or receptacle, and hermetically closed. Burney and Pemberton (2016, 29) argue that Gross treated traces as significant in their contextuality, as evidence of a crime scene, not principally focusing on their own materiality in relation to identification and comparison. However, my primary sources on Dutch criminalistics show that the examination of hair did revolve around the notion of identity. Already in 1881, a textbook of forensic medicine in the Dutch East Indies mentioned hair, alongside teeth, skin, height, tattoos, and scars, as indicators of personal identity, when this could not be established on the basis of witness statements or clothing and needed to be established from race, nationality, or personality. Microscopic examination of hair was mentioned as an important indicator. The author, Dr. Schneider, wrote that the size and shape of hair differed per race, age, gender, and the place on the body. He provided examples of the measurements of, e.g., female pubic hair and male beard hair. He also mentioned that the shape of the roots of the hair differed. He gave instructions on how to compare the dry hair of the suspect with the dry hair found on the hands of the victim or on bloody murder weapons. The whole hair, up to the roots, had to be examined using the right lighting. Then the procedure had to be repeated with wet hairs (Schneider 1881, 104, 169–171). So, this scientist regarded hair as an indicator of race, age, and gender.

In his textbook for forensic doctors working in the Dutch East Indies from 1912, Hermanus Frederik Roll (1912, 140–143) mentioned hair in his section on crime traces, stating that, since most people in the Dutch East Indies had black hair, the examination of hair would be less useful than in Europe. The second edition of this textbook, dating from 1918, testified to the development of the new science of criminalists and included many more images, also of hair. Hair was mentioned in the section on wounds and tears: the way hair stuck to the skull could be of information regarding the way the body had died. The physician should carefully inspect the hairs on the body with a loupe, cut them, and save them for microscopic examination. Lesions of hairs could also lead to the unraveling of the crime (Roll 1918, 184–185). In the section on trace evidence, drawings of men's and women's hair, of different colors, were shown, as well as a photo of an axe to which the victim's hair was stuck (Roll 1918, 270–271). In this edition, too, the lesser value of the microscopic inspection of hair in the East Indies was mentioned, since the majority of people there had black hair and the differences between individuals were supposed to be minor. The microscopic examination not only served to determine the identity of the hair but also to decide whether the hair had fallen out, been pulled, cut (usually men had cropped hair, whereas women's hairs had intact ends), or abraded (e.g., in hairs on body parts covered in clothing or marked by sweat). Hair was very important as trace evidence, Roll (1918, 272–273) repeated, but its study needed a lot of expertise. Here, hair was mostly seen as an indicator of racial or gender identity, providing information on the perpetrator but also on the features of the crime.

In court cases, as well, scientists examining hair were called in as expert witnesses from around 1900. They, for instance, established connections between hair found in the blood left on the murder weapon and hair found on the coat of the victim (Case Gerard Vial 1901). In a Dutch sexual assault case from 1904, hair was examined under the microscope. Two apothecaries examined the traces on clothing, hat, brooch, and head hair. On the female victim's brooch they found a piece of light-blonde hair with a root on one end. Its average thickness, the lack of a clearly visible canal, and the strangely scaly surface were great similarities with the light-blond hairs of the suspect. The hairs of the victim were darker blonde, had a smooth surface, and a clearly visible canal. For comparison, the hairs of the fur hat were also examined, which showed completely different hallmarks, different from human hair. The scientists concluded there was no similarity between the hair found in the brooch and the head hair of the woman. In the final verdict the experts were mentioned extensively. The court believed that the hair showed similarities in thickness and color with that of the suspect, especially since the abnormalities of his hair were considered rare (Case Harm Dikken 1904). So, identity here revolved around the differences between humans and animals and differences between human beings, although the exact, unique identity could not be established.

To conclude, in the first decades of the twentieth century, forensic science emphasized the use of hair as trace evidence to establish the identity of the killer and to reconstruct the crime. Gender, race, and the difference between humans and animals could be important, but hair could never be a unique identifier, such as fingerprints. The symbolic meanings of hair, forwarded by anthropologists, are absent here. Modern criminalists stripped hair of its many ritual, magic, and fetishistic meanings. And yet, hair, as part of the criminal's body, was not only disciplined by science. Following Deleuze, we might say that hair forms part of assemblages that include other objects and persons at the crime scene, for instance, connecting blood, axe, perpetrator, and victim. These assemblages give hair its meaning. Thus, hair and the body had the potential to take several forms according to the assemblages they were part of.

Women Punished by Hair Shaving After the Second World War

The twentieth century would see a revival of older meanings of hair. Hair as a symbol of femininity and sexuality returned during and after the Second World War. The Nazis shaved their prisoners' heads to dehumanize them, the loss of hair depriving especially women prisoners of their individual identity and worth (Pergament 1999, 49). Directly after the Second World War, in several European countries, girls' and women's hair was publicly cut or shaved as a form of punishment for allegedly sleeping with German soldiers. Fabrice Virgili has analyzed the *tontes* (shearings) in France, correcting many established notions. Virgili argues, for instance, that some men were shaved as punishment, too. More importantly, he states that women were accused of several forms of collaboration. The shearings were well-organized public assertions of patriotic unity. They were partly an effort to wipe out traces of the enemy, hence a form of purification, sometimes meant to channel violence. Hair shearing was regarded as a form of humiliation and desexualization of women. It expressed contempt for women, who functioned as scapegoats to expunge the anger and guilt of the French people, reaffirming French virility. Collective shame forced women back into the private sphere (Virgili 2004).

Virgili's historical-anthropological analysis also delves into the symbolic meanings of hair. He argues that shaving women's hair was not a punishment for sexual relations with the Germans but a gendered punishment for collaboration. Only later did it gain the sexual connotation in the public imaginary (Virgili 2004, 56). Hair was a symbol of femininity; the longer the hair, the guiltier the woman was. Hair was also a metaphor for the sexual body that had been culpable of sleeping with the enemy. Women were thus regarded as the seducers (German soldiers not being punished). By cutting their hair, the French crowds desexualized and defeminized these women, thereby reappropriating their bodies, especially since they were (partially) nude during the hair cutting. The sadistic and voyeuristic elements of this ritual made it into a virtual rape (Virgili 2004, 235–237).

In the Netherlands, many Dutch girls and women were shaved, too, possibly following the French example. However, these actions were not organized "top down" but seem to have been spontaneous "people's courts." Rianne Oosterom argues that, at least in Utrecht, the majority of townspeople disapproved of the treatment of these *moffenhoeren*

(Germans' whores). Still, in an article supporting the shearings, the communist resistance newspaper *De Waarheid* wrote that hair was "the greatest ornament for women, but it was also the greatest defamation to lose it" (quoted in Oosterom 2013, 10). The shearing of hair was clearly meant to take away female dignity. Danish historian Anette Warring (2006, 89, 120) states that this was already a recognized way of punishment in Europe. Warring adds that it was also a symbolic castration of women: their sexuality was taken away, thus diminishing their powers of attraction. It was done out of jealousy and moral objections, but also because of hurt national pride (women's bodies were seen as national possessions). Nevertheless, Warring warns against interpreting the cutting off of hair

> too rigidly as a symbolic act of punishment which refers to, and can be understood primarily on the basis of, an underlying cultural system. Rather than interpreting it as a cultural sign in the semiotic sense, it should instead be seen as a social strategy or practice deployed to obtain something. By cutting the hair . . . not only her appearance but also her relations to society were altered. The punishment was visible and for a certain duration of time it would bear witness to her treason. It was a punishment of the body that had been given to the enemy, and as such it was a sexualised retribution for a sexual act.
>
> (2006, 120)

Warring adds that the reason why the assailants chose this particular method of punishment was not explained explicitly at the time. She states that the method was not invented for the occasion but neither stemmed from a deep-rooted cultural tradition. Although women's hair had been targeted before, as a punishment for infidelity or fraternizing with strangers, other methods of punishment had been used as well (Warring 2006, 120). Nevertheless, the type of punishment does remind us of early modern dishonoring punishments: just like adulteresses, then, in 1945, in at least one Dutch town, only the hair of *married* women who had had intercourse with German soldiers was cut (Diederichs 2006, 170). Moreover, the women's heads were shaved and often poured over with pitch or red lead; sometimes a swastika was carved onto the head. A French underground newssheet from 1942 advocated the shaving of the heads of women who had given their bodies to the Germans, adding "you will be whipped, and on all your foreheads the swastika will be branded with a red hot iron" (Virgili 2004, 95; Diederichs 2006, 174). This reminds us very much of early modern corporal punishment, with the only difference that these brandings were not permanent if they were done with paint or in the remaining hair. Warring describes the women in these cases as being "branded like cattle" (2006, 121). The animal metaphor underlines the association of bald women with animals. We can find a similar association in a text by the Dutch author Jan Wolkers, who witnessed the cutting of girls' hair after the war in Oegstgeest: "When she was completely bald and pulled off the chair she stood with closed eyes and her hands pressed against her temples as a defenceless larva or fetus" (quoted in Diederichs 2006, 70). Not only women's sexuality was taken from them but also their humanity. I would like to refer back to anthropologist Hallpike's theory on hair, which associates hair with being outside of society and with animality, and the shaving of the hair with rejoining society. I would argue that both aspects apply to the women whose heads were shaved after the Second World War, yet maybe not completely in the way that Hallpike meant. Whereas for Hallpike, long hair equals being outside of society and animality, here it is the shaved women who are treated like animals and who are pushed out of society. At the same time, the ritual as such is meant to purify society and to make the people as a whole regroup.

Conclusion

The early modern hair cutting was strongly connected to shame and gender. In the modern period, with the rise of sciences like criminal anthropology, anthropology, and psychiatry, hair was increasingly used as indicator of normality and abnormality, as Herzig has shown. It was thus also a means of classification (relating to race, gender, or criminality). The rise of forensic science around 1900 focused solely on hair as a means of identification, of determining the perpetrator, rather than as a unique identifier. Forensic scientists distinguished between human and animal blood stains, and textbooks of criminalistics also classified hair on the basis of species, race, and gender. What is striking is that early forensic science regarded hair as stripped from all its symbolic connotations: hair does not refer to the self or soul, or to sexuality, castration, power, or dirt. It hardly belongs to the body anymore: it is one of the "silent witnesses," one of the material traces on the crime scene.

It could be argued that forensic science's focus on identification and classification nevertheless contributed to disciplining the body of criminals. This disciplining, however, features much more prominently directly after the Second World War, when the heads of many girls and women were shaved as punishment. Here, the symbolical value of hair, relating to gender and sexuality, returns. Hair is here also strongly connected to being human, whereas the women without hair are described as "cattle" or "larvae." The role of hair as marking the human-animal divide is missed by most anthropological theorists of hair. This shows how many meanings hair may have. In this sense, hair can never be disciplined or pinned down: it is always becoming and growing, full of potential connotations. It forms assemblages with other persons and objects and acquires meaning from the specific cultural context.

References

Berg, Charles. 1951. *The Unconscious Significance of Hair*. London: Allen & Unwin.

Bisbing, Richard E. 1982. "The Forensic Identification and Association of Human Hair." In *Forensic Science Handbook*, edited by Richard Saferstein, 184–221. Englewood Cliffs, NJ: Prentice Hall.

Bourke, Joanna. 2011. *What It Means to Be Human: Reflections from 1791 to the Present*. Berkeley: Counterpoint.

Buchanan, Ian. 1997. "The Problem of the Body in Deleuze and Guattari: Or, What Can a Body Do?" *Body & Society* 3 (3): 73–91.

Burney, Ian, and Neil Pemberton. 2016. *Murder and the Making of English CSI*. Baltimore: Johns Hopkins University Press.

Case Gerard Vial. 1901. "North Holland Archives Haarlem." *Archive Court of Justice Amsterdam*. Inv. no. 226.

Case Harm Dikken. 1904. "North Holland Archives Haarlem." *Archive Court of Justice Amsterdam*. Inv. no. 249.

Cole, Simon A. 2001. *Suspect Identities: A History of Fingerprinting and Criminal Identification*. Cambridge, MA: Harvard University Press.

Deleuze, Gilles. 1997. "Desire and Pleasure." Translated by Melissa McMahon. Accessed on October, 28. www.artdes.monash.edu.au/globe/delfou.html

de Win, Paul. 1991. *De schandstraffen in het wereldlijk strafrecht in de zuidelijke Nederlanden van de middeleeuwen tot de Franse tijd bestudeerd in Europees perspectief*. Brussels: Paleis der Academiën.

Diederichs, Monika. 2006. *Wie geschoren wordt moet stil zitten. De omgang van Nederlandse meisjes met Duitse militairen*. Amsterdam: Boom.

Douglas, Mary. [1966] 2008. *Purity and Danger: An Analysis of Concept of Pollution and Taboo*. London/New York: Routledge.

Foucault, Michel. [1975] 1995. *Discipline & Punish: The Birth of the Prison*. New York: Vintage Books.

Franke, Herman. 1990. *Twee eeuwen gevangen, Misdaad en straf in Nederland*. Utrecht: Het Spectrum.

Geltner, Guy. 2014. *De gesel en de ander: lijfstraffen en culturele identiteit van Oudheid tot heden*. Amsterdam: Amsterdam University Press.

Hallpike, Christopher Robert. 1969. "Social Hair." *Man* 4 (2): 256–264.

Helps, Lisa. 2007. "Body, Power, Desire: Mapping Canadian Body History." *Journal of Canadian Studies* 41 (2): 126–150.

Herzig, Rebecca M. 2015. *Plucked: A History of Hair Removal*. New York: New York University Press.

Horn, David. 2003. *Lombroso and the Anatomy of Deviance*. New York: Routledge.

Hunt, Lynn. [2007] 2008. *Inventing Human Rights: A History*. New York: W. W. Norton & Company.

Leach, Edmund Ronald. 1958. "Magical Hair." *The Journal of the Royal Anthropological Institute of Great Britain and Ireland* 88 (2): 147–164.

Maes, Louis. 1947. *Vijf eeuwen stedelijk strafrecht: bijdrage tot de rechts-en cultuurgeschiedenis der Nederlanden*. Antwerp: De Sikkel.

Mak, Geertje, and Saskia Bultman. 2019. "Forms of Identity: Paper Technologies in Dutch Anthropometric Practices around 1900." *The International Journal for History, Culture and Modernity*, 7: 64–109.

Martin, Rudolf. 1914. *Lehrbuch der Anthropologie in systematischer Darstellung mit besonderer Berücksichtigung der anthropologischen Methoden für studierende Ärzte und Forschungsreisende.* Jena: G. Fischer.

Monballyu, Jos. 2003. "Heksen, hun buren en hun vervolgers in de Leiestreek: Een sociale benadering van de heksenprocessen te Olsene en Dentergem in 1660–1670." *Handelingen van de Maatschappij voor Geschiedenis en Oudheidkunde te Gent* 57: 121–182.

Ofek, Galia. 2009. *Representations of Hair in Victorian Literature and Culture.* Aldershot: Ashgate.

Oosterom, Rianne. 2013. "Geknipt voor de vijand. Mentaliteit en mening in bevrijd Nederland over het kaalscheren van 'moffenmeiden.'" BA thesis, Utrecht University.

Pergament, Deborah. 1999. "It's Not Just Hair: Historical and Cultural Considerations for an Emerging Technology." *Chicago-Kent Law Review* 75 (1): 41–58.

Roll, Hermanus Frederik. 1912. *Leerboek der Gerechtelijke Geneeskunde.* Vol. 1. The Hague: Algemeene Landsdrukkerij.

Roll, Hermanus Frederik. 1918. *Leerboek der Gerechtelijke Geneeskunde voor de scholen tot opleiding van Ind. artsen.* Vol. 1. 2nd edition. The Hague: Martinus Nijhoff.

Sachs, Hans. 1997. "History of Hair Analysis." *Forensic Science International* 84 (1–3): 7–16.

Schneider, Dr. Fr. 1881. *Catechismus der Gerechtelijke Geneeskunde voor Nederlandsch Indië.* Soerabaija: Gebr. Gimberg & Co.

Schreuder, Willem. 1949. *Eerste optreden op de plaats van een misdrijf.* Leiden: A.W. Sijthoff.

Silverman, Lisa. 2001. *Tortured Subjects: Pain, Truth, and the Body in Early Modern France.* Chicago, IL: The University of Chicago Press.

Synnott, Anthony. 1987. "Shame and Glory: A Sociology of Hair." *British Journal of Sociology* 38 (3): 381–413.

Virgili, Fabrice. 2004. *La France "virile." Des femmes tondues à la Libération.* Paris: Payot & Rivages.

Warring, Anette. 2006. "Intimate and Sexual Relations." In *Surviving Hitler and Mussolini: Daily Life in Occupied Europe*, edited by Roberta Gildea, Olivier Wieviorka, and Anette Warring, 88–128. New York: Berg.

Watson, Katherine D. 2011. *Forensic Medicine in Western Society: A History.* New York: Routledge.

9 Citizen to Convict

The Consumption of the Body in the Age of Prisoner Reentry

CalvinJohn Smiley

Introduction

Prison changes the body. The US criminal justice system incarcerates more than two million bodies per year and more than 650,000 of those bodies are released each year. In other words, the American prison system is a convoluted system that cycles thousands of bodies in and out of its labyrinth annually. Penal institutions serve both a symbolic and literal representation of what can be done to the body. The former relies on *deterrence* to dissuade individuals from engaging in acts deemed illegal. The latter serves as a place of *incapacitation* to hold individuals who have engaged in acts considered unlawful. Therefore, the fundamental purpose of prison is to restrict the body. This constraint on the body[1] occurs in visible and invisible, physical and emotional, and tangible and abstract manifestations. I argue that the body goes through various changes and labels, moving from "citizen" to "convict" to "ex-con." Utilizing historical texts, academic scholarship, and media representations, this chapter will focus on the transition from "convict" to "ex-con" and the ways that the prison experience informs the body upon release.

Prisoner reentry is simply the transition of the body from confinement to community. However, while simplistic as it may seem, reentry in the United States comes with complicated, complex, and fragile obstacles and barriers that strip legal rights such as voting and social relationships with family. Therefore, it is unlikely that the body comes out of prison unscathed, and reentry is not the culmination but rather an extension of control over the body. Furthermore, in the United States, incarcerated bodies are overwhelmingly racially Black, low-income, and from urban communities (Uggen, Manza, and Behrens 2003; Pettit and Western 2004; Abu-Jamal and Fernández 2014). Consequently, it is important to investigate the history of racialized punishment in the United States. In other words, racism in the United States has played a pivotal role in how law enforcement is used to control the Black body.

In this chapter I examine how prisoner reentry informs the body. First, I discuss a brief history of punishment, specifically on the Black body in the United States. Throughout American history, the Black body has been consumed by White Supremacy for economic, political, and social profit through systems such as chattel slavery and convict leasing. In this section, I outline the various ways labor, punishment, politics, and sexuality were used to control the Black body. Secondly, I explore the exponential growth of the US prison system, particularly a shift from public (seen) to nonpublic (unseen) displays of punishment. Here, I will discuss how prisons modify the body, particularly how these institutions are designed to create environments of tense violence. Hence, the prison setting has a profound and lasting impact on the body, beyond the prison walls. Third, this chapter looks at how those lasting impacts manifest into different burdens that inform the returning body as consequences of being incarcerated. In particular, understanding the visible and invisible, the physical and emotional, and the tangible and abstract ways prison and reentry configure the body. While I recognize that human agency is an important component to the body, this chapter focuses on the ways structural inequalities and punishments are exacted on the body. The body is often a source of resistance (Middlemass and Smiley 2016a), however, forms of resistance are beyond the scope of this chapter. Finally, in order to grasp the concept of what punishment does to the body, I look toward prison abolition to examine what the body needs to be healed and protected.

History of Punishment

Punishment and the body have a symbiotic relationship. Various civilizations, ancient and modern, have an association with using some form of violence on the body, including torture and death. Prior to the Age of Enlightenment, many acts deemed criminal were thought to be the work of demons that took over the human body. However, early criminologists such as Cesare Beccaria (1797), utilizing the scientific method, believed criminality was a learned behavior. Beccaria argued that individuals have free will to choose to commit a criminal act. Therefore, in order to prevent criminality, the fear of punishment must be incorporated into society and for those who break the law, punishment must be perceived to be severe, certain, and swift in order to deter future criminal actions (Beccaria 1797).

Historically, punishment was a spectacle. Michel Foucault (1979) describes, in detail, the torture and death of Robert-François Damiens, who was publicly executed via the method of drawing and quartering in eighteenth-century France after being accused of attempted regicide. James Whitman (2003) argues that degradation plays a pivotal role in how societies punish and carry out sentences. In other words, to simply punish without announcement would not have the desired effect on the masses. Therefore, public degradation is equally important because it frames society's relationship with the accused offender. Durkheim ([1895] 2007) contends that crime is a functional aspect of society, as it creates social cohesion, sets the standards of right and wrong, and, most importantly, creates jobs. However, over time, with the birth of modern prisons, public forums have been replaced with nonpublic settings. In the early nineteenth century, the Pennsylvania and Auburn prison models were created (James 2014). Both institutions demanded prisoners remain completely silent and utilized solitary confinement as forms of punishment. This was to foster repentance through the belief that criminal behavior could be unlearned. Prisons were designed with the idea of reform. However, it did not take long for prisons, even with the best of intentions, to become violent and harmful spaces. Early research on these institutions found that solitary confinement created both physical and mental illness (James 2014). In order to maintain these spaces of complete obedience, brutality was inflicted on prisoners. In the earliest known memoir by a Black prisoner, Austin Reed describes his imprisonment in both the juvenile and adult prison institutions in New York in the mid-nineteenth century. Reed states, "He [Superintendent] then tied my hands around the post, saying to the inmates that he wanted them all to take warning by the punishment which I was to receive for making my escape, and hoped that it might be a lesson to them hereafter" (Reed 2016, 39). Additionally, modern prisons perfected surveillance, introducing the model which Jeremy Bentham (1843) called the "panopticon," where one individual could oversee all the prisoners from a central location. Ultimately, prisons became the standard punishment in American society.

American punishment cannot be divorced from the institution of chattel slavery. The earliest known records of African slaves date back to 1619, when 19 individuals were brought to the shores of the United States. The practice of legal slavery lasted until 1865, only being abolished following the American Civil War. During this roughly 250-year period, the Black body was private property. While the institution of slavery is not unique, American bondage relied on racial segregation based on pseudo-scientific arguments of race being a fixed identity set by nature. In other words, racial differences created biologically different species, which was used to reinforce the separation of the races and justify the practice of human bondage. In addition, American slavery was a paternalistic system that created an infrastructure of White Supremacy. In order to do this, a conscious effort of stripping African culture from the enslaved was enforced. This idea of inferiority of African (Black) people was spread throughout the Americas. The third president of the United States, Thomas Jefferson, expounded and sought to define those racial differences in his work *Notes on the State of Virginia*. He writes, "I advance it therefore as a suspicion only, that the blacks, whether originally a distinct race, or made distinct by time and circumstances, are inferior to the whites in the endowments both of body and mind" ([1787] 1997, 103). Jefferson's philosophy, which he situates in a scientific argument, is only reinforced by legal status of Black bodies. In the landmark decision of *Scott v. Sanford*, the Supreme Court ruled in 1857 that the Black body could not be considered a citizen. Chief Justice Roger Taney stated, "In the opinion of the court, the legislation and histories of the times, and the language used in the Declaration of Independence, show that neither the class of persons who had been imported as slaves nor their descendants, whether they had become free or not, were then acknowledged as a part of the people, nor intended to be included in the general words used in that memorable instrument" (1857). He thus, once again, reaffirmed the position of the Black body as inferior and not a part of American society.

During this time, discipline was used on the Black body to reinforce the practices of slavery. The whip became one of the most infamous tools wielded by slave masters. Frederick Douglass (2002), a former slave who escaped, discusses his time under the duress of Mr. Covey, an exceptionally brutish man who was known as a slave breaker and who would destroy the body and mind. Angela Davis (2003) describes the ingenious ways slave discipline and punishments were *gendered*. In her book *Are Prisons Obsolete?*, Davis recounts the slave narrative of Moses Grandy, who describes how pregnant slaves were made to lie on the ground with their stomach positioned in a hole to protect the unborn fetus, or rather preserve future labor, subsequently putting profit over human dignity. Even after emancipation, exploitative servitude continued because the Thirteenth Amendment of the US Constitution has a clause that states, "Neither slavery nor involuntary servitude, except as a punishment for a crime whereof the party shall have been duly convicted, shall exist within the United States, or any place subject to their jurisdiction" (Browne-Marshall 2010). In other words, the continued practice of bondage continued but instead of calling the subjugated "slave," they are now "criminal."

The practice of convict leasing began prior to the end of slavery; however, it rapidly grew after the Civil War. The Jim Crow system emerged to suppress newly freed Black people from being viewed as equal through a variety of Black codes such as laws of moral turpitude, vagrancy, public drunkenness, loitering, or gathering in groups. In *Slavery by Another Name*, David Blackmon (2009) illustrates the ways in which law enforcement, the courts, corrections, public institutions, and private businesses profited from this system of forced labor in the name of criminal justice. During this time, infrastructure such as roads, rails, and bridges were built by convict labor. In addition, private companies used convict labor for coal mining and timbering. This type of harsh work and horrendous conditions caused physical ailments, spread of disease, and death. If a convict refused to work, they were disciplined in various manners, from whipping to loss of food.

Interestingly, while slavery and convict leasing used brutal disciplinary measures on the Black body, they were in some ways guided by different economic incentives. Under slavery, the slave was private property and therefore had an intrinsic value to the owner, who could use or lease their labor for profit. In other words, the slave held just as much, if not more, value than the commodity it procured or produced. Under these circumstances, the slave body was punished for punitive purposes with death being a last resort rather than primary goal. However, under convict leasing, Black bodies were now citizens because of the Fourteenth Amendment of the US Constitution. Black citizens went from property to competition for commodities and resources. Under the leasing system, the Black body was state property and the convict was not what held any essential value; it was simply the labor they procured or produced. The incentive was now to keep the bodies flowing into the system. In his book *Worse Than Slavery*, David Oshinsky, quoting LG Shiver, describes Parchman Farm, which was a slave plantation converted into a prison: "The convict's condition was much worse than slavery. The life of the slave was valuable to his master, but there was no financial loss . . . if a convict died" (1996, v). Death was a common occurrence during convict leasing, whether from harsh work conditions, brutal discipline, or rampant disease and malnutrition.

Under slavery and convict leasing the Black body was consumed and exploited. As illustrated above, the Black body was used for work and labor purposes. In order to maximize this effort, brutal methods of punishment were thrust upon the Black body. However, beyond work and punishment, the Black body was exploited in various other ways. Politically, the Black body was used to maximize Southern votes in Congress in what became known as the Three-Fifths Compromise of 1787 (Browne-Marshall 2010). During the Constitutional Convention, a debate about Southern representation and taxes spurred the notion that slaves could be counted as three-fifths of a person, which bolstered the population of Southern states giving more delegate seats in the House of Representatives. Under this condition, the notion of Black bodies being sub-human was negotiated to give some level of humanity to maximize White Supremacy. This legacy of using captive bodies for political purposes still exists today. In many states, incarcerated individuals are counted in the US Census where they reside rather than where they are from (Levine 2018). Therefore, when local, state, and federal budgets are allotted to towns, cities, counties, and districts, areas are profiting off bodies that are only in their community because of their confinement and this money is not being used to benefit those incarcerated.

Besides political exploitation, sexual consumption was a primary use of slaves and imprisoned laborers. Instances of rape were rampant throughout slave plantations. Frederick Douglass, among other well-known former slaves, was the product of the White owner raping a Black slave. The film *12 Years a Slave* follows the autobiography of Solomon Northup, a Black man who was kidnapped and sold into slavery. The film highlights the vicious sexual relationship the White owner has with his Black female slaves. Beyond the heteronormative prose surrounding rape culture within slave narratives, Vincent Woodard's (2014) book *The Delectable Negro* highlights homoeroticism, sexual assault of male slaves, and human consumption. Woodward, using historical slave texts, highlights the various ways homoeroticism played out within slave culture in both figurative and literal ways. In the former, how Black bodies were sexualized and exploited, while in the latter, the need for Black labor to produce capital, as well as the consumption and practice of cannibalism of Whites eating Black bodies. He stresses how homoeroticism permeated forms of discipline and punishment in slave culture. He describes how slaves were stripped and whipped while naked or forced to stand exposed on auction blocks to be inspected by potential White buyers. David Blackmon (2009) also describes similar practices of stripping the Black body naked for discipline during convict leasing. Other forms of torture, such as refusal of food, clothing, or shelter, all deform and change the body. Blackmon describes the various methods of securing Black bodies on large plantations, which included the "ball and chain" affixed to the leg of a convict or instances of individuals being hog tied to a pole and forced to sleep outside. In the film *Django Unchained*, the slave girl, Broomhilda, is punished for disobeying her master by being placed naked in a metal box under the hot Southern sun. Moreover, practices of sexualized violence have not escaped modern prisons. Angela Davis (2003) describes the ways incarcerated women are subject to various forms of physical and sexual violence in the name of "security" through practices such as anal and vaginal cavity searches. In addition, both men and women who are incarcerated receive inadequate health services and have higher health risks (Johnson 2018). For example, in many American states, pregnant women are chained to their beds during childbirth (Roberts 2017). Experts in the field of obstetrics and gynecology have indicated that this policy could have dire health risks to both the mother and child (Sichel 2008). Political prisoner and former death row inmate Mumia Abu-Jamal (2009) highlights that various US military personnel who were indicted for torture in the infamous Abu Ghraib prison camp were Pennsylvania correctional officers. Abu-Jamal indicates that many of the complaints of torture and sadistic treatments by the same individuals arrested for torture of Muslim detainees fell on deaf ears. The Black and Brown body has, and still remains, a place of forced labor, punishment, sexual exploitation, experimentation, and political resource. The next section highlights the rise of mass incarceration, which has led to exponential growth in reentry.

Mass Incarceration

Coming out the Civil Rights Era, the United States had passed landmark legislation such as the Civil Rights Act of 1964, the Voting Rights Act of 1965, and the Fair Housing Act of 1968. In addition, the Supreme Court ruled unanimously in favor of the *Loving v. Virginia* case that found anti-miscegenation laws unconstitutional. Federally, under President Lyndon B. Johnson, the United States began what became known as the "War on Poverty," which sought to eradicate illiteracy by providing better educational opportunities as well as create better healthcare for all American citizens (Hinton 2016). These steps were only made possible because of the work of Civil Rights activists who pressured federal legislators into action.

The seemingly progressive strides of this movement were halted in 1968 after the presidential election of Richard M. Nixon, who campaigned on "law and order." Exploiting fears of civil unrest, particularly in Northern urban cities where uprising had occurred, such as Detroit, Michigan, and Newark, New Jersey, Nixon vowed to his constituents that he would restore the moral fabric of American values through making criminal justice a top priority. Much of the rhetoric Nixon espoused was coded language that became synonymous with more traditional racial views of White Supremacy. Recently, a Nixon aide admitted that many of the policies that were implemented during his administration targeted Black Americans and other counterculture movements, such as Hippies (LoBianco 2016). Therefore, tough-on-crime measurements replaced the social justice cause and the "War on Poverty" became the "War on Crime." This shift in national discourse permeated down to the state level. In 1973, New York Governor Nelson Rockefeller passed the first set of mandatory minimum sentencing guidelines for drug offenders (Gonnerman 2004). Under mandatory minimums, offenders would have to serve a specific amount of time before being eligible for release, which circumvented prosecutorial and judicial discretion. Jennifer Gonnerman (2004) examines the life of Elaine Bartlett in her book *Life on the Outside*, and the way mandatory minimum sentences impacted her and her family. Bartlett was arrested for transporting a small amount of cocaine from New York City to upstate New York, where she was caught, tried, and convicted, and received a 20-year-to-life sentence. The fact that Bartlett had no prior criminal history did not matter. During the second half of the twentieth century, both state and federal legislation began passing punitive laws and harsh sentencing guidelines such as "three strikes" laws and "truth-in sentencing" procedures. Beyond drug laws, policies surrounding all types of criminal behaviors that are known as "street" crimes (e.g., murder, assault, robbery) received harsher guidelines. In 1976, the Supreme Court reinstated the use of capital punishment in the case *Gregg v. Georgia*. Previously, in 1972, the Supreme Court had suspended the use of capital punishment in its ruling of *Furman v. Georgia*. Punitive, but more so retributive, punishment became part of the legal culture moving into the twenty-first century.

By 2000, there were over 1.3 million individuals incarcerated at the state and federal level in the United States (Beck and Harrison 2001). The US prison system saw a 700 percent increase from 1970 to 2005 (Austin, Naro, Fabelo 2007) and, by 2009, there were over 2.4 million individuals incarcerated or under parole supervision, with another four million formerly incarcerated individuals in society (Schnittker, Massoglia, and Uggen 2011). The Pew Center released a report in March 2009 indicating that one out of every 31 Americans was under some form of criminal justice supervision (Warren et al. 2009). David Garland (2001) refers to this exponential growth as mass imprisonment, known colloquially as "mass incarceration." Loic Wacquant (2010) disputes the term "mass" but refers to this as more of "hyper" incarceration. Wacquant makes this distinction because the concentration of who is incarcerated in the United States is neither random nor representative of all citizens, but in fact targeting specific populations, namely Black Americans. Wacquant (2005) highlights that in America, Young + Black + Male can have lethal consequences if one does not know their "place" or is considered "out-of-place." Trayvon Martin, a 17-year-old Black male, was perceived to be "out-of-place" by a neighborhood watchman, who ultimately killed him. In recent years, with the proliferation of social media and smartphone devices, the deaths of unarmed Black males have been captured, documenting these deaths. However, in order to justify these killings, law enforcement and media outlets have posthumously portrayed these individuals as criminals, which extends the legacy of the Black body being portrayed as a "brute" or "thug" (Smiley and Fakunle 2016). This idea of blackness being synonymous with suspicion and, ultimately, criminality is highlighted in the disproportionate rate of Blacks being stopped, questioned, and frisked. A report produced by Delores Jones-Brown (2013) highlights the unequal amount of stops of Black and Latino young men by the New York Police Department. In addition, the US Justice Department (2017) released reports on Ferguson, Missouri, and Baltimore, Maryland, following the deaths of two unarmed young Black men, Michael Brown and Freddie Gray, respectively, indicating wide ranges of discriminatory bias based on race. In short, the Black body has been overrepresented and policed in the criminal justice system based on an ideology that has perpetuated the notion that Black bodies are inherently more criminal.

Beyond Black males, Black women have also been impacted by a bias system. Matthew Desmond argues that housing discrimination, particularly in the form of eviction, impacts Black women in greater rates than other racial groups. Desmond argues, "If incarceration has become typical in the lives of men from impoverished black neighborhoods, eviction has become typical in the lives of women from these neighborhoods" (2012, 91). The forced movement of the Black body has lasting and devastating impacts on familial and social networks. Even still, Black women have not avoided incarceration and are becoming the fastest growing prison population (Frazier 2016). Natalie Sokoloff writes about the impacts of Black female incarceration, stating, "The vast majority of women in prison are mothers with children under the age of 18 (70 percent). . . . With just over one-quarter (28 percent) of children of incarcerated mothers being cared for by their fathers" (2003, 36). Reminiscent of the slave auctions, incarceration separates families with the physical and emotional removal of the mother from children and the family.

Prisons by design and practice are spaces of hyper-violence. While the original purposes set out in the nineteenth century were to separate individuals so that they could repent and seek forgiveness, this is not how prisons operate. Prisons are often overcrowded places that function in a state of viciousness, which perpetuates fear, anxiety, and stress. Often times, correctional staffs are purveyors of this ferocity. In California's maximum-security prison, Corcoran State Prison, guards created a "gladiator days" fighting club, where prisoners were forced to fight (Cherney 2015). The case of Kalief Browder highlights much of the violence that occurs in American jails and prisons. Browder was arrested at age 16 and held at New York City's Riker's Island jail pending trial. Because Browder's family could not afford bail, he remained on the island for over three years. During that time, fellow prisoners, as well as correctional officers, attacked Browder. Ultimately, his case was dismissed and all charges dropped. However, this did not mean that Browder's time incarcerated did not have an impact on his life after prison. Sadly, two years after his release, Browder committed suicide (Gonnerman 2015). He had attempted suicide previously, all stemming from his incarceration on Riker's Island. Browder's case, along with many others, highlights the deep impact that prison has on the body. Individuals go from being labeled a "convict" to "ex-con" upon release. While reentry is the removal of the body from restrictive walls, this does not mean that reentry is absent of the altered body. The following section discusses how the body is transformed because of incarceration in the reentry process in several ways, including visible and invisible; physical and emotional; and tangible and abstract.

Reentry and the Body

The prison body is made through a set of rituals and customs that ensue in penal environments, which includes fighting, stabbing, and other assaults that occur frequently and regularly. The body must adapt to this total institution (Goffman 1968), which tries to diminish agency over the self. In the end, the prison experience does not stop at the prison gates but ultimately extends beyond prison walls and into the reentry process.

The prison body is inscribed (Moran 2012) by markers of time while incarcerated. It develops in *visible* and *invisible* manifestations. Much of the visible representations of prison are shown on the body. This could include several indicators. Scars showcase the visible representation of violence in prison settings. Weapons such as shanks and razors are accessible and slicing a victim can cause scarring, particularly on the face. The term "buck fifty" refers to being slashed across the face, typically stretching from ear to mouth (Tong, McIntyre, and Silmon 1997). This type of injury leaves the victim with a lifelong brand of the violence they endure. Other such visible markers of prison are that of chipped or missing teeth (Moran 2012). Often times, losing teeth are results of either fighting or lack of dental care. In either scenario, tooth loss impacts the body and recognition of the face. Without teeth or the proper amount of teeth, one's smile is changed, which could influence certain anxieties such as embarrassment as well as inability to eat certain foods. Beyond teeth, prison tattoos like scars tell a narrative of the body (Moran 2012). Improvised tattoo guns make tattooing accessible in prison. These mostly crude designs can narrate an individual's prison journey, such as the amount of time they have been incarcerated or where they have been incarcerated; they convey ideologies (e.g., White Supremacist tattoos) or remember loved ones such as a child's name tattooed on one's arm (Rozycki Lozano et al. 2011). These artistic expressions are meant to remain on the body well past the prison experience and aid as reminders of one's time imprisoned. Finally, access to clothing upon leaving prison serves various points in the ability to gain entrance and acceptance back into society, particularly conveying a certain look or identity for the body (Smiley and Middlemass 2016).

Contrary to the visible markers are the invisible signs of being incarcerated. In fact, the unseen is often times much harder to reconcile and come to terms with because it cannot be placed or measured. In regard to many of the invisible markers is the stigma and label of being formerly incarcerated, known as an "ex-con." This title carries a negative connotation and the individual cannot untie him or herself from their previous experiences in life. This label can impact one's own identity in how they see themselves and manifest into social behaviors of self-fulfilling prophecy (Merton 1948). Devah Pager's (2008) scholarship highlights the disparities and stigma Black men face post-incarceration in seeking employment. Often times, the invisible is neglected, downplayed, or dismissed, either consciously or unconsciously. In these cases, the invisible injuries of incarceration are not fully fleshed out, particularly the various traumas that are witnessed. Beyond the notion of the harm that could be inflicted on the body, one has to acknowledge how being a witness to violence could have a lasting impact on a person. Mika'il DeVeaux (2013) discusses the horrendous violence he witnessed while incarcerated and how many of these images have remained with him over the years, even though he was not directly involved.

Moving from the visible and invisible dichotomy are the *physical* and *emotional* pains that are inflicted on the body because of incarceration. Physical injury does not land solely on the ideas of violence but on the way that time changes the body (Middlemass and Smiley 2016b). Inadequate hygiene in prison environments limits access to haircuts, makeup, lotion, and feminine products, which impact the body's look, feel, and representation, as do signs of premature aging such as hair loss, arthritis, and the need for glasses. Prison cells are often small and shared with other occupants, limiting mobility as well as reducing natural light. In the *Autobiography of Malcolm X* by Alex Haley ([1965] 1992), Malcolm X discusses his eyesight changing while incarcerated. He states, "I had come to prison with 20/20 vision. But when I got sent back to Charlestown [prison], I had read so much by the lights-out glow in my room at the Norfolk Prison Colony that I had astigmatism and the first pair of eyeglasses that I have worn ever since" (1992, 218). The lack of quality food impacts an individual's diet. Spanos (2013) discusses the use of "nutral-oaf" that is often fed to prisoners and the health impacts this mash of various ingredients has on the body. Furthermore, research indicates that roughly 38.5 percent of federal prisoners, 42.8 percent of state prisoners, and 38.7 percent of persons in jail suffer from chronic conditions such as diabetes, hypertension, and asthma (Wilper et al. 2009). These conditions have the potential of being debilitating or even life-threatening without proper medical care.

Emotional changes are often unseen and harder to understand. Research indicates that the prison experience can cause various forms of stress and anxiety (Buckaloo, Krug, and Nelson 2009; Boothby and Clements 2000). Moreover, research has looked at links between incarceration and post-traumatic stress disorder (PTSD; Punamäki, Qouta, and Sarraj 2010; Hutton et al. 2001). Raymond Santana, a member of the Central Park Five,[2] stated in an interview, "When I was released, I was released in 1995, and I couldn't get a job. I didn't know how to function in society because there was no transitional programs that take me from prison to the streets" (2012). The lack of preparedness sent Santana back to prison, as he became involved with drug distribution to try and earn an income and cope with the time he spent incarcerated for a crime he did not commit. These emotional changes impact mental health and the prison experience can give someone overactive awareness of their surroundings or desensitize an individual to the point where they lack emotional awareness.

The last way that the prison changes the body is through the *tangible* and *abstract* binary. In this concept, both of these ideas are recognized by the notion of citizenry. For example, the majority of individuals who have been incarcerated experience some level of disenfranchisement (Manza and Uggen 2008). In some cases, one might lose the right to vote while incarcerated, while others might lose this right indefinitely. Therefore, this shapes the way the body is treated post-incarceration. The idea of voting is an abstract concept. It lends itself to concepts of democracy and freedom. However, the act of voting is tangible. In this instance, the ability to go to a polling station, enter a polling booth, and pull a lever for a candidate is a physical act that is exercised via the right of citizenry.

Consequently, "voting" is both an abstract notion and tangible action that is reserved for individuals with full citizenry. Hence, the post-prison body is thrust into this dilemma of losing certain legal rights such as the right to vote. This then puts to question the idea of citizenry and whom these rights protect. If democratic values of suffrage are important tools of a so-called democratic state, then why limit certain individuals from carrying out this right? In essence, the post-prison body is still paying a premium price for their conviction. No longer is it in the tangible act of imprisonment but in the abstract notion of freedom that is essentially confined. Under this premise, persons who have been incarcerated are not full citizens, or rather only part of their body is acceptable and the other remains outside the purview of the state.

Conclusion

Prison changes the body. Yet, this change in the American context has a much more linear and historical background in which it is tethered, specifically, to the Black body. Throughout the American experience, beginning with the age of exploration, to colonialism, imperialism, and now neoliberal policy, control and manipulation of the Black body is an important tool of White Supremacy. In fact, without control over the Black body, White Supremacy loses its grasp. Prisons are used to control Black bodies and maintain White Supremacy. Prisons signify the physical representation of holding the body but symbolize breaking the spiritual, mental, and emotional traits that are embodied. Prisons are places of both physical and symbolic violence that do not practice rehabilitation but rather focus on retribution.

If one looks at prisons as problematic spaces that damage both individuals and communities, reforms are not the answer and abolition must become the focus. Abolition is not just a lofty idea of a utopian society but a willingness to engage in very difficult and uncomfortable discourse about what to do with those who have, in some cases, engaged in violent acts or other actions deemed socially irresponsible. Abolition places an emphasis on early intervention and implementing policy that focuses on securing affordable and safe housing, equitable educational opportunities, adequate and universal healthcare, and restorative justice to repair injuries in society. Since 95 percent of all persons incarcerated are released (Travis, Solomon, and Waul 2001), a much-needed revision of justice must occur. In other words, the vast majority of those who go into the gallows come out and we, as a society, must be ready to heal and protect both victims *and* offenders, ultimately moving away from the current prison model to a much more progressive and justifiable model that keeps the body intact, both in the physical and nonphysical dimension.

Notes

1. It is important to understand that the body encompasses both the physical apparatus but also includes the mind and spirit.
2. The Central Park Five were five Black and Latino teenagers accused, tried, and convicted of the rape of a White female jogger in New York City and ultimately exonerated by DNA evidence. For further detail, see Natalie Byfield's book, *Savage Portrayals: Race, Media and the Central Park Jogger Story.*

References

Abu-Jamal, Mumia. 2009. *Jailhouse Lawyers: Prisoners Defending Prisoners v. the USA.* San Francisco: City Lights Books.

Abu-Jamal, Mumia, and Johanna Fernández. 2014. "Locking Up Black Dissidents and Punishing the Poor: The Roots of Mass Incarceration in the US." *Socialism and Democracy* 28 (3): 1–14.

Austin, James, Wendy Naro, and Tony Fabelo. 2007. *Public Safety, Public Spending: Forecasting America's Prison Population 2007–2011.* Washington, DC: The Pew Charitable Trust, Public Safety Performance Project.

Beccaria, Cesare. 1797. *On Crimes and Punishment.* Translated by H. Pallouci. Indianapolis: Hackett Publishing.

Beck, Allen J., and Paige M. Harrison. 2001. "Prisoners in 2000." *Bureau of Justice Statistics, US Department of Justice.* Accessed on July 17, 2018. www.bjs.gov/content/pub/pdf/p00.pdf

Bentham, J. 1843. *The Works of Jeremy Bentham, vol. 4 (Panopticon, Constitution, Colonies, Codification).* Liberty Fund, Inc. Accessed on July 17, 2018. http://oll.libertyfund.org/titles/1925

Blackmon, Douglas A. 2009. *Slavery by Another Name: The Re-Enslavement of Black Americans from the Civil War to World War II.* New York: Anchor.

Boothby, Jennifer L., and Carl B. Clements. 2000. "A National Survey of Correctional Psychologists." *Criminal Justice and Behavior* 27 (6): 716–732.

Browne-Marshall, Gloria J. 2010. *The U.S. Constitution: An African American Context.* 2nd edition. New York: Law and Policy Group Press.

Buckaloo, Bobby J., Kevin S. Krug, and Koury B. Nelson. 2009. "Exercise and the Low-Security Inmate: Changes in Depression, Stress, and Anxiety." *The Prison Journal* 89 (3): 328–343.

Byfield, Natalie P. 2014. *Savage Portrayals: Race, Media, and the Central Park Jogger Story.* Philadelphia: Temple University Press.

Cherney, Max. 2015. "When Prison Guards Force Inmates to Fight." *Vice*, April 3. www.vice.com/en_us/article/av45x5/when-prison-guards-force-inmates-to-fight-403

Davis, Angela Y. 2003. *Are Prisons Obsolete?* New York: Seven Stories Press.

Department of Justice. 2017. *Federal Reports on Police Killings: Ferguson, Cleveland, Baltimore, and Chicago.* Brooklyn, NY: Melville House.

Desmond, Matthew. 2012. "Eviction and the Reproduction of Urban Poverty." *American Journal of Sociology* 118 (1): 88–133.

DeVeaux, Mika'il. 2013. "The Trauma of the Incarceration Experience." *Harvard Civil Rights-Civil Liberties Law Review* 48: 257–277.

Douglass, Frederick. 2002. "Narrative of the Life of Frederick Douglass (1845)." In *The Classic Slave Narratives*, edited by Henry Louis Gates, Jr., 323–436. New York: Signet Classic.

Durkheim, Émile. 2007. "The Rules of Sociological Method (1895)." In *Classical and Contemporary Sociological Theory: Text and Readings*, edited by Scott Appelrouth and Laura Desfor Edles, 95–102. Thousand Oaks: Pine Forge Press.

Foucault, Michel. 1979. *Discipline and Punish: The Birth of the Prison*. Translated by Alan Sheridan. New York: Vintage.

Frazier, Charise. 2016. "Here Is Why Women of Color Are the Fastest Growing Jail Population." *NewsOne*, August 18. https://newsone.com/3511585/women-of-color-are-the-fastest-growing-jail-population/

Garland, David, ed. 2001. *Mass Imprisonment: Social Causes and Consequences*. New York: Sage.

Goffman, Erving. 1968. *Asylums: Essays on the Social Situation of Mental Patients and Other Inmates*. New Brunswick: AldineTransaction.

Gonnerman, Jennifer. 2004. *Life on the Outside: The Prison Odyssey of Elaine Bartlett*. New York: Picador.

Gonnerman, Jennifer. 2015. "Kalief Browder, 1993–2015." *The New Yorker*, June 7. www.newyorker.com/news/news-desk/kalief-browder-1993-2015

Haley, Alex. [1965] 1992. *The Autobiography of Malcolm X as Told by Alex Haley*. New York: Ballantine Books.

Hinton, Elizabeth. 2016. *From the War on Poverty to the War on Crime*. Cambridge: Harvard University Press.

Hutton, Heidi E., Glenn J. Treisman, Wayne R. Hunt, Marc Fishman, Newton Kendig, Anthony Swetz, and Constantine G. Lyketsos. 2001. "HIV Risk Behaviors and Their Relationship to Posttraumatic Stress Disorder among Women Prisoners." *Psychiatric Services* 52 (4): 508–513.

James, Kirk A. 2014. "The History of Prisons in America." *Medium*, November 18. https://medium.com/@kirkajames/the-history-of-prisons-in-america-618a8247348

Jefferson, Thomas. [1787] 1997. "The Difference Is Fixed in Nature." In *Race and the Enlightenment: A Reader*, edited by Emmanual Chukwudi Eze, 95–103. Malden, MA: Blackwell Publishing.

Johnson, Lauren. 2018. "Silent But Deadly: Hepatitis C and Prison." *Pittsburgh Courier*, February 7. https://newpittsburghcourieronline.com/2017/07/19/silent-but-deadly-hepatitis-c-and-prison/

Jones-Brown, Delores D., Brett G. Stoudt, Brian Johnston, and Kevin Moran. 2013. *Stop, Question, and Frisk Policing Practices in New York City: A Primer*. New York, NY: Center on Race, Crime and Justice, John Jay College of Criminal Justice.

Levine, Sam. 2018. "2020 Census Will Continue to Count Prisoners Where They Are Incarcerated." *HuffPost*, February 8. www.huffingtonpost.com/entry/2020-census-prison-population_us_5a7cb966e4b044b3821b0507

LoBianco, Tom. 2016. "Report: Aide Says Nixon's War on Drugs Targeted Blacks, Hippies." *CNN*, March 24. www.cnn.com/2016/03/23/politics/john-ehrlichman-richard-nixon-drug-war-blacks-hippie/index.html

Manza, Jeff, and Christopher Uggen. 2008. *Locked Out: Felon Disenfranchisement and American Democracy*. New York: Oxford University Press.

Merton, Robert K. 1948. "The Self-Fulfilling Prophecy." *The Antioch Review* 8 (2): 193–210.

Middlemass, Keesha M., and CalvinJohn Smiley. 2016a. "Jumpsuit to Button-Down: Clothing Used as Resistance in Prisoner Reentry." *Journal of Criminal Justice & Law Review* 5 (1–2): 63–80.

Middlemass, Keesha M., and CalvinJohn Smiley. 2016b. "Doing a Bid: The Construction of Time as Punishment." *The Prison Journal* 96 (6): 793–813.

Moran, Dominique. 2012. "Prisoner Reintegration and the Stigma of Prison Time Inscribed on the Body." *Punishment & Society* 14 (5): 564–583.

Oshinsky, David. 1996. *Worse Than Slavery: Parchman Farm and the Ordeal of Jim Crow Justice*. New York: Free Press.

Pager, Devah. 2008. *Marked: Race, Crime, and Finding Work in an Era of Mass Incarceration*. Chicago, IL: University of Chicago Press.

Pettit, Becky, and Bruce Western. 2004. "Mass Imprisonment and the Life Course: Race and Class Inequality in US Incarceration." *American Sociological Review* 69 (2): 151–169.

Punamäki, Raija-Leena, Samir R. Qouta, and Eyad El Sarraj. 2010. "Nature of Torture, PTSD, and Somatic Symptoms among Political Ex-Prisoners." *Journal of Traumatic Stress* 23 (4): 532–536.

Reed, Austin. 2016. *"The Life and Adventures of a Haunted Convict,"* edited by Caleb Smith, New York: Random House.

Roberts, Dorothy. 2017. *Killing the Black Body: Race, Reproduction, and the Meaning of Liberty*. 20th Anniversary edition. New York: Vintage Books.

Rozycki Lozano, Alicia T., Robert D. Morgan, Danielle D. Murray, and Femina Varghese. 2011. "Prison Tattoos as a Reflection of the Criminal Lifestyle." *International Journal of Offender Therapy and Comparative Criminology* 55 (4): 509–529.

Santana, Raymond. 2012. "Member of 'Central Park Five' Talks Justice." *Tell Me More NPR*, November 15. www.npr.org/2012/11/15/165214082/justice-for-the-central-park-five

Schnittker, Jason, Michael Massoglia, and Christopher Uggen. 2011. "Incarceration and the Health of the African American Community." *DuBois Review* 8 (1): 1–9.

Sichel. Dana L. 2008. "Giving Birth in Shackles: A Constitutional and Human Rights Violation." *American University Journal of Gender, Social Policy & the Law* 16 (2): 223–255.

Smiley, Calvin John, and David Fakunle. 2016. "'From 'Brute' to 'Thug': The Demonization and Criminalization of Unarmed Black Male Victims in America." *Journal of Human Behavior in the Social Environment* 26 (3–4): 350–366.

Smiley, Calvin John, and Keesha M. Middlemass. 2016. "Clothing Makes the Man: Impression Management and Prisoner Reentry." *Punishment & Society* 18 (2): 220–243.

Sokoloff, Natalie. 2003. "The Impact of the Prison Industrial Complex on African American Women." *Souls* 5: 31–46.

Spanos, Alexander J. 2013. "The Eighth Amendment and Nutraloaf: A Recipe for Disaster." *Journal of Contemporary Health Law & Policy* 30 (1): 222–248.

Taney, Roger. 1857. *Dred Scott v. Sanford 60 U.S. 19 How. 393 (1857)*. www.law.cornell.edu/supremecourt/text/60/393

Tong, Virginia, Tom McIntyre, and Herman Silmon. 1997. "What's the Flavor? Understanding Inmate Slang Usage in Correctional Education Settings." *Journal of Correctional Education* 48 (4): 192–197.

Travis, Jeremy, Amy L. Solomon, and Michelle Waul. 2001. *From Prison to Home: The Dimensions and Consequences of Prisoner Reentry*. Washington, DC: Urban Institute.

Uggen, Christopher, Jeff Manza, and Angela Behrens. 2003. "Felony Voting Rights and the Disenfranchisement of African Americans." *Souls* 5 (3): 48–57.

Wacquant, Loïc. 2005. "Race as Civic Felony." *International Social Science Journal* 57 (183): 127–142.

Wacquant, Loïc. 2010. "Class, Race & Hyperincarceration in Revanchist America." *Daedalus* 139 (3): 74–90.

Warren, Jennifer, Susan Urahn, Richard Jerome, Jake Horowitz, and Joe Gavrilovich. 2009. *One in 31: The Long Reach of American Corrections*. Washington, DC: Pew Research Center on the States.

Whitman, James Q. 2003. *Harsh Justice: Criminal Punishment and the Widening Divide between America and Europe*. New York: Oxford University Press.

Wilper, Andrew P., Steffie Woolhandler, J. Wesley Boyd, Karen E. Lasser, Danny McCormick, David H. Bor, and David U. Himmelstein. 2009. "The Health and Health Care of US Prisoners: Results of a Nationwide Survey." *American Journal of Public Health* 99 (4): 666–672.

Woodard, Vincent. 2014. *The Delectable Negro: Human Consumption and Homoeroticism within US Slave Culture*. New York: New York University Press.

Part V
The Entangled Body

10 Aesth/Ethical Bodies

Bracha Ettinger's *Eurydices* and the Encounter With the Other's History

Anna Kisiel

> I am bound to others before being tied to my body.
> —Emmanuel Lévinas (1991, 76)

Bodies Entangled in History

The photograph of naked women and children awaiting their execution, taken in 1942 in the Mizocz ghetto, forms the background for Bracha L. Ettinger's most famous painting series, entitled *Eurydice*. Covered with layers of paint, the figures standing in a row in the original photograph become almost invisible; yet, these canvases tend to reveal the fragments of their bodies entangled in tragic historical events. In the *Eurydices*, Ettinger—who is an artist, psychoanalyst, feminist, matrixial theorist, and member of the Second Generation after the Holocaust—provides us not only with a testimony to the women's trauma but first and foremost with an artistic project aiming at its affective embodiment. Ettinger's artworks are constantly interweaving with her matrixial theory based on the assumption that separation, castration, and binary oppositions are not the only paths toward subjectivity; inspired by the feminine bodily specificity, she proposes that, in its origin, subjectivity is a result of an encounter between two or several becoming subjects that are not necessarily known to each other but nevertheless intimately connected.

In this chapter, I will endeavor to prove that the (female) body is a site and source of an ethical transhistorical encounter with the anonymous Other(s). In light of this thesis, the aim of my chapter is twofold. Firstly, I wish to juxtapose Emmanuel Lévinas with Bracha L. Ettinger in order to delineate the ethical aspect of the body in her matrixial theory while emphasizing Ettinger's indebtedness to and dialogue with Lévinasian humanism. Secondly, I will attempt to identify and interpret the ethical dimension of corporeality in Ettinger's chosen artistic pieces— *Eurydice*, No. 17, *Eurydice*, No. 37, and two untitled sketches sharing the Eurydicean motif—keeping in mind that art in the Ettingerian frame is inextricably linked to the intrauterine existence; precisely, art might offer a humanizing pathway to the fragmented memory of this state. Through this slightly affective reading moving toward the limits of representation, I will try to show how these artworks interweave with and contribute to the given theoretical stances.

Linkages and Reciprocities

From the biological viewpoint, the body is a *sui generis* container for the womb placed within it. This organ is an essential part of the motherly body, but it by no means implies that women are defined by its very presence—or possession; still, as Ettinger notes, "anatomy makes a difference that we should open to conceptualization" (2006c, 181). The existence of the womb within the female corporeality—which is the womb's "*heimlich*" space—provides us with a possibility of theorizing the body itself. Built on the notion of the *matrix*, which is the prenatal signifier of non-phallic feminine difference,[1] Ettinger's theory endeavors to broaden the possibilities of Freudian and Lacanian psychoanalysis by means of including femininity and female body within this field. Similarly to the function the male bodily organ serves in classical psychoanalysis, the female body becomes a model for theorizing subjectivity formation; therefore, Ettinger rejects the threat of essentialism or biological determinism. Regarding the questions of "nature," female specificity, and difference, Ettinger writes:

> The incestuous *in/out-side* relation (*rapport*) between subject-to-be and archaic-m/Other-to-be, by its connection to female corporeal invisible specificity (which is the place where this incest takes place), is the source in the Real for a matrixial stratum. This source should not mislead us into seeking the matrixial encounter in biological nature, any more than the phallic structure stands for the corpo-Real male sexual organ (although it is related to it). . . . In the matrix, her sex difference in terms of female bodily specificity, and experiencing an affected linking to that specificity (the Real), inscribes a paradoxical sphere on the Symbolic's margins.
>
> (2006b, 105, emphasis in the original)

At this point, the notion of incest ought to be clarified. In the matrixial context, this term gains a new meaning. Ettinger notes that in the prenatal phase, the desire to establish a linkage with the Other—felt by both partners in the encounter—is an ordinary phenomenon, essential to the emergence of life and to the orienting to the matrixial sphere (see Ettinger 2006a, 88; Ettinger 2006b, 94). Therefore, instead of being forbidden, the incestuous relation becomes humanizing and creative. In this excerpt, Ettinger makes it clear that even though the said meeting between two becoming subjects is held within the feminine specificity (and thus becomes the origin of the matrixial), the matrix itself is no more natural than the phallus, grounded upon the male organ. Moreover, female connectedness to her corporeality contributes to the movement toward the peripheries of the Symbolic: the order Ettinger expands in her thought.

As it is the body that becomes a space abundant in linkages, in this respect the matrixial theory connotes Emmanuel Lévinas's take on ethics, in which corporeal connotations seem to resurface time and again. As early as *On Escape* (published in French in 1935)—his reexamination of Martin Heidegger, (embodied) self, and ego—Lévinas ponders upon the connection between physical conditions, including malaise and nausea, and the eponymous evasion, which is described as the urge to "*break that most radical and unalterably binding of chains, the fact that the I [moi] is oneself [soi-même]*" (2003, 55, emphasis in the original). Bodily tropes continue in Lévinas's *oeuvre*, returning also in *Totality and Infinity*. They can be found, among others, in the notion of sensibility: "the *mode* of enjoyment" (1969, 135, emphasis in the original)—not to be mistaken for representation and not related to understanding—which is available to the body (see 1969, 136–137). We read: "One does not know, one lives sensible qualities: the green of these leaves, the red of this sunset. . . . Sensibility, essentially naïve, suffices to itself in a world insufficient for thought" (1969, 135).[2] Neither rational nor intuitive, the way proposed by Lévinas affirms an affective and sensual encounter without objectification, without the firm division into the *I* and the *non-I* and yet entirely egoistic (see 1969, 134, 187–188). The question of the body in the concept of sensibility gains in importance and visibility in *Otherwise than Being*; this book also offers a more straightforward affirmation of the Other in sensibility. Being *for* the Other is absorbed into a greater pre-subjective fundamental stratum, which—although not derived from cognition—turns out to be strikingly corporeal (1991, 76–77). Because of its non-cognitive—or rather pre-cognitive—status, this stratum is not necessarily preoccupied with the issue of selfhood; as Lévinas writes, "I am bound to others before being tied to my body" (1991, 76). He goes on to claim that "subjectivity is sensibility—an exposure to others, a vulnerability and a responsibility in the proximity of the others, the-one-for-the-other" (1991, 77). These excerpts reveal Ettinger's entanglement in Lévinas's ethical reflections, considering that in Ettingerian psychoanalysis the body provides a site of an originary encounter with the Other.

What is, then, the position that the female/motherly body occupies in Lévinasian thought? Kathryn Bevis undertakes this issue by means of analyzing two metaphors used by the philosopher: maternity and dwelling. In her interpretation of the excerpts from *Totality and Infinity*, she notes: "Woman is the precondition for human reflection because she represents . . . a primary human contact and sociality which is not yet the transcendent, shattering presence of the face-to-face relationship with the Other" (2007, 321; see Lévinas 1969, 154–155). Simultaneously, she argues, the female here is neither dialogic nor personalized; not being a part of the discourse, a subject, or an Other, she functions as a hospitable envelope for someone else's selfhood (2007, 321). In turn, in *Otherwise than Being*, the status of the maternal body undergoes transformation. In his revised definition of sensibility, Lévinas utilizes maternal metaphors to grasp the complexity of the ethical relationship, which is based on extreme responsibility that assumes the option of being affected, or even hurt, by the Other (see Lévinas 1991, 75). Maternity—the site of bearing and the first habitation, by means of which one is originally "bound to others"—becomes the primary, sensible structure of relations.

These questions are also tackled by Lisa Guenther in her analysis of the feminization/maternalization of Moses in Lévinas. She stresses that in the Lévinasian reading of the Book of Numbers and the figure of Moses present there, one does not have to be a mother in a biological sense to act *like* one.[3] The author notes that using Moses as a maternal figure leads to a number of ethical implications concerning responsibility, substitution, politics, and justice. Guenther concludes that an encounter with the Other makes one become "a unique, embodied, and responsible self" (2006, 131), despite one's gender, identity, social status, or biological qualities. Motherhood understood in such a way is freed from these bounds, becoming instead the mode of responding to the Other's ethical demand (Guenther 2006, 132–133).

When it comes to the issues of connectedness, encounter, and maternal body, Ettinger's indebtedness to Lévinas can be easily spotted. However, when it comes to femininity itself—leaving for a moment its motherly aspect—Ettinger clarifies that for the philosopher it becomes an impassable limit. In *Existence and Existents*, Lévinas proclaims that "the other *par excellence* is the feminine" (1978, 85, emphasis mine).[4] Ettinger notes the paradoxical image arising from the writings discussed above: the woman lacks the dialogic quality and is Otherness *per se*, and yet the originary difference is undoubtedly feminine, as feminine/motherly attributes are ascribed to it. Moreover, femininity is absent in Lévinas's late work. Ettinger puts forward a hypothesis that this notion has been abandoned not so much because it has ceased to be essential from the ethical viewpoint as the philosopher has started to comprehend the fact that the woman is not an absolute Other: that, instead, the feminine informs the very notion of subjectivity. She clarifies that the attributes of subjectivity are precisely the traits that used to be identified as feminine (2006c, 190). These assumptions are confronted in a conversation between the two theorists, in which Lévinas makes a diagnosis that

> Woman is the category of future, the ecstasy of future. It is that human possibility which consists in saying that the life of another human being is more important than my own, that the death of the other is more important to me than my own death, that the Other comes before me, that the Other counts before I do, that the value of

the Other is imposed before mine is. . . . The feminine is that differ-ence, the feminine is that incredible, unheard of thing in the human by which it is affirmed that *without me the world has meaning*.
(Lévinas in conversation with Ettinger 2006,
142–143, emphasis in the original)

In this passage, we can see to what an extent Lévinas's vision of the feminine coincides with his ethical postulates. Although he claims that femininity is yet to come, the qualities that resurface in this quotation—being for the Other, responsibility and encounter—prove that in Lévinas's thought the woman is persistently present despite her seeming absence.

Ettinger's take on femininity posed in the context of Lévinas consoli-dates his position as a precursor of the ethical aspect of the matrixial theory. As she claims, femininity is responsible for a change in the under-standing of the subject, channeled toward a humanizing encounter (see 2006c, 190). The encounter—directly linked to the feminine corporeal specificity—is preceded by and contains an act of self-fragilization, nec-essary to face the Other openly despite the threat of suffering. Most significantly, Ettinger strongly objects to treating the woman as a total Other. She argues that in the matrixial reading of Lévinasian femininity, responsibility changes into *response-ability*, which, while still including the activities of taking care of the Other and answering the Other's calls, also adds the possibility of the actual responding: a human(e) dialogue and asymmetrical reciprocity, missing in this philosopher's proposition (see 2006c, 190).

What helps Ettinger establish her position beyond the limitations faced by Emmanuel Lévinas is the shift to the border-Other, linked to the notion of severality. Using weaving metaphors, Ettinger describes the female as a border-Other, with whom relations can be established pro-vided that "we follow upon *her* threads in the texture and the textile of the web" (2006c, 194, emphasis in the original). She continues: "She is weaving and being woven. She bears witness in the woven textile and tex-ture of psychic transsubjectivity" (2006c, 196). These excerpts illustrate the matrixial structure of connections, which is active-passive, recipro-cal, and asymmetrical. Responsive and willing to share, the matrixial woman is also a witness (see 2006c, 198). However, the condition of her potential response and generosity of sharing is eagerness to pursue the traces which belong not to her only and yet can be found within her psychic space. Emphatically, the imagery utilized here distinguishes femi-ninity from fusion or symbiosis; that is, instead of borderless fluidity, it is seen as a web comprised of threads and strings. Nevertheless, Ettinger stresses that "matrixial subjectivity does not mean an endless multiplicity of singular individuals, but rather a limited multiplicity—a severality—that traverses subjectivity" (2006c, 196). Being a notion modeled upon motherly specificity and prenatal/pregnancy phase, severality makes any subject a co-subject, whereas an Other—in spite of gender assigned to it—ceases to be total because of its intimate proximity to the *I*.

In her theory, Ettinger transcends Lévinasian intersubjectivity, which, despite being directed toward the Other, remains immersed in singularity and individual experience. Simultaneously, by no means does she reject the prominence of his proposition, placing the female body at the center of his ethics. Interestingly enough, while for Lévinas "the other *par excellence* is the feminine," for Ettinger it is subjectivity that *par excellence* is the feminine. Moreover, the originary subjectivity resurfacing in Lévinas's writings, described by means of female attributes, corresponds to the matrixial proposition of trans- or co-subjectivity that transcends the premode of subjectivization. That which serves the purpose of deconstructing an individual subject in the Ettingerian stratum is motherhood: a primary structure and source of relations to be found in both theories. Importantly, all the notions described here reveal their eminent entanglement in corporeality and embodiment. Ettinger's recognition of femininity as the ethical subject itself moves us to the future Lévinas has spoken of.

The notions of weaving, connectedness, reciprocity, and co-subjectivity are inextricably linked to Ettinger's claim that the feminine corporeality can generate and carry knowledge; this, in turn, calls to mind Lévinasian ethics, which renders the maternal body the origin of signification. As Ettinger maintains, the female ought to be open and ready to reconnect with her matrixial stratum of severality in order to find meaning in the traces of experiences originating there. To be precise, "[s]he must uncognizantly know her *non-I*(s)" (2006d, 142, emphasis in the original). This excerpt emphasizes that the knowledge about the border-Other(s) is not cognitive, and yet it is relevant for the matrixial sphere, being simultaneously its aim and its condition—the subject both strives for it and needs to be receptive and fragilized during its acquisition. What is more, it is the female that makes a further transfer of such knowledge—or rather "sub-knowledge" (Ettinger 2006d, 142)—possible as she passes it on to the subjective stratum, on whose margins it is supposed to reside, challenging the phallic organization but still remaining side by side with it.[5] In his ethical reading, Lévinas links the body to signification, posited before language and yet comprehensible. Using the metaphor of motherhood, he describes the workings of signification by means of caretaking activities (1991, 77). Moreover, he reveals the interrelatedness of subjectivity, sensibility, and signification as follows: "[S]ubjectivity is sensibility—an exposure to others, a vulnerability and a responsibility in the proximity of the others, the-one-for-the-other, that is, signification" (1991, 77). This excerpt again shows the dialogic relation between Ettinger's system and Lévinas's thought, as the main qualities of the matrixial stratum of subjectivization are fragility and fragilization, response-ability, and closeness aiming at opening oneself for the Other and his or her non-cognitive knowledge. Finally, Lévinas notes: "Subjectivity of flesh and blood in matter—the signifyingness of sensibility, the-one-for-the-other itself—is the preoriginal signifyingness that *gives sense, because it gives*" (1991, 78, emphasis mine). Hence he establishes the role of maternity and its connection not only to sensibility, but also to sense and signification. The maternal-like body becomes the source of meaning precisely because it has a capacity for providing and sharing. Therefore, the intersection of these two approaches depicts the body—be it feminine, maternal, or any body—as an originary locus and a pathway of knowledge beyond the linguistic system. Strictly corporeal and nonlinguistic, this kind of knowledge also goes beyond history itself. In its rereading of the feminine body, Ettinger's psychoanalysis provides the space for experiencing the *non-I*'s pain and trauma—and thus reembodying them—which becomes particularly significant while considering the Holocaust. At this exact point, ethics, art, and (shareable) history meet.

Aesth/Ethical Meetings

Historically speaking, the women from the Mizocz ghetto are abandoned; yet, are they completely alone? The image they are captured in is a result of the anonymous photographer's gesture of dubious ethical value. They were murdered in the name of terrible collective responsibility: on 13 October 1942 there was a revolt of prisoners in the Mizocz ghetto, Ukraine, the day after which all the men, women, and children were executed one by one (approximately 1,700 people). In the picture, the women's bodies are naked: they are humiliated and exposed to the voyeuristic gaze, left with no chance to defend themselves. Bracha L. Ettinger's art can be claimed to change their hopeless position. *Eurydice*, No. 17 (1994–1996)[6] is one of Ettinger's early works in the series, in which the women are still discernible.[7] The surface of the piece is blurry and grainy; the bright background merges with black and purple shades. The photographic frame the artist works on includes the most characteristic and recurring face of the series, located in the middle of the canvas. We can observe the women with no difficulty, but they are not exposed, being partly clothed by means of Ettinger's artistic actions, as the grain and the color hide their bodies from the voyeur's look. These females are not alone in a threefold sense. At the moment they are captured in the image, they are in "collectivity," as Deleuze and Guattari would put it, supporting and warming each other, waiting for their shared fate. Years later, they encounter the artist, who compassionately witnesses and works through their pain. Finally, as they are pronounced "Eurydices," they also encounter the viewer, who, like Orpheus, simultaneously sees them dead and keeps them alive.

Not only are the Eurydices not alone, but also are they hospitable, "inviting" to their canvas Ettinger's mother and father from the prewar photo taken in the street of Łódź in 1936. In *Eurydice*, No. 37 (2001),[8] the background determines the border between two temporalities, two fates, two stories, and disparate mental and physical states. The left side reveals the trace of the posed photograph of young, possibly careless, joyful people—Bluma Fried and Uziel Lichtenberg, Ettinger's parents-to-be. We cannot see them clearly because of the technique that employs pigment, ashes, and dust, yet their shapes are easy to recognize. Their faces, in turn, merge with the canvas. The right side is inhabited by the face already encountered in the previous painting. Even though it is blurry, composed of smears of black paint, we seemingly can read more from it than from Ettinger's parents' invisible expression. Here, we may discover fear and shock of this anonymous woman. The right side, therefore, is occupied by the victim—one of anonymous females, who is about to die. On the left we watch the future survivors, who during the war fled Poland, escaped from several ghettoes, camps, and countries, to finally reach Palestine (see Zegher and Pollock 2012, 249). What we, viewers, witness is an encounter beyond these differences: an encounter embodied on one canvas.

Embodiment takes its literal form in *No Title-Sketch* (1988–1989),[9] which, to put it bluntly, is "crowded" with bodies. This time, it is not the background that enacts the separation; the contrast between the two realities is instead achieved by the juxtaposition of naked bodies of women standing in a row (a different photographic frame than in the works analyzed above) with elegantly dressed people. The faces of Bluma and Uziel are sharper than in *Eurydice*, No. 37, and there is an illusion that they are looking toward the females on the right. Here, the two groups are facing each other, unable to turn back. Sentenced by the artist to this co-existence, they are challenged to survive the aesthetically eternalized moment of fragility. The sketch becomes a space of interweaving, proximity, and blurred borders; because of the unbearably embodied presences it hosts, it opens a lane toward an ethical relation, in which Otherness is always already partial.

Another *No Title-Sketch*, produced in 1985,[10] provides us with yet another manifestation of the analyzed motif. The technique is the same, but the effect appears to be entirely different because of the painting's space being dominated by the color purple. The artwork has three main sets. The upper left part reveals a visible frame from the Mizocz photograph showing the returning face of a woman. Here, we can observe who surrounds her: behind her there is a woman with a baby in her arms and another woman in front of her—a little girl who, as we can see in the original, non-manipulated photograph, is holding tight yet another female, maybe her own mother. This girl reappears in a close-up on the right, just next to Ettinger's parents. They, in turn, are standing in the middle of the sketch, as if in the foreground, overlaying the crowd. Despite dark colors, the image reveals more than the previously described ones. Maybe one of the reasons is that this sketch is made in 1985, thus being one of Ettinger's early works, created seven years before she started the first *Eurydice* painting (1992–1994). Later in her art we can note the nonlinear, yet proceeding disappearance of the origin photo. Still, what we as viewers observe here is more than the Barthesian "return of the dead" (Barthes 1981, 9) in the medium of photography. It also at least endeavors to go beyond Susan Sontag's claim that the great number of images of atrocity we encounter makes us more immune to the horror they depict (see Sontag 1979, 19–21). Ettinger's aim is not to immunize the spectator; rather, by means of hosting the naked bodies—already dead but still alive, depending on the chosen temporality—the image calls us to gaze and to respond, posing an ethical demand in a Lévinasian sense.

The artworks have been presented in a non-chronological manner not without purpose; the aim of such an arrangement was to show that the origin photographs' invisibility is in perpetual motion, whether we look at Ettinger's works individually or if we analyze them as a series of interconnected images engaged in a dialogue. When we focus on the bodies of women from Mizocz, we note that they are in no way explicit or straightforward; nor are they easily accessible for the spectator. Ettinger's artistic technique includes the processes of covering the photograph, cropping it, veiling and unveiling certain fragments of bodies or faces, to name a few. All these actions lean toward de-othering and de-objectifying these women, that is, resisting voyeurism, scopophilia, or erotization they may be or might have been subject to. Importantly, it cannot be said that they are disappearing as a sacrifice for the Other, as in the Lévinasian take on vulnerability. Rather, in an Ettingerian manner, they are "partial[ly] disappearing to allow joint-ness" (Ettinger 2006d, 145), becoming vulnerable so as to let the Other approach them. As a result, when their Other—the viewer—in his or her fragility reaches the space they occupy, he or she is called not to leave but to remain and co-exist. The spectator is demanded to become a Moses figure, who faces that which is unintelligible and potentially unbearable but nevertheless carries the burden that was assigned to him or her. Through their partial invisibility, the female bodies—of women, daughters, mothers, grandmothers, girls, pregnant women—invite us to become one of them, without appropriation or objectification, but in terms of being interwoven, joining their affective web in a struggle toward humanity.

When it comes to the alliance between the Mizocz Eurydices and Bluma Fried and Uziel Lichtenberg, we might choose to stick to the interpretation that what we witness in these works is the meeting of personal and historical trajectories; after all, there is a picture from Ettinger's family album and a drastic photographic document of the genocide. Yet, it is more complex than that. Born to a Jewish family, Ettinger was never able to meet the majority of her relatives, which is far from being a marginal issue for her. In one of her notebooks, we read about the photograph from Mizocz:

> I want her to look at me! That woman, her back turned to me. The image haunts me. It's my aunt, I say, not, my aunt's the other one, with the baby. The baby! It could be mine. What are they looking at? What do they see? I want them to turn toward me. Once, just once. I want to see their faces. . . . Please look at me once. You are my dead aunt, or you are my living aunt or you are someone I [had] known. . . . Mother-I, my aunt could have been my daughter.
>
> (Ettinger 1993, 67)

It has not been confirmed whether Ettinger's relatives were in the Mizocz ghetto, and whether one of the women might have been Ettinger's aunt. These quotations shatter the binary opposition between the private and public spheres, which outwardly merge here; in other words, they disturb the simplicity of the meeting that seemed to take place between two groups of people, anonymous to each other, having different fates but linked by the fact of being victims of the Holocaust. However, it is not the point, for these excerpts are not aimed at revealing the historical connection between Bracha L. Ettinger and the Mizocz women, which would somehow explain her so-called "interest" in the case. Instead, from the Ettingerian viewpoint, historical knowledge does not play a role once one enters the matrixial stratum. As I tried to show, such a feminine connection is made possible thanks to the maternal-female bodily specificity. In Ettinger's painting—which continuously interlaces with her theory—corporeality is significant not *per se*, but because it takes one to the level of the matrixial sphere of an almost-boundless proximity. An encounter with the bodies of Eurydices becomes trans-historically ethical, notwithstanding the anonymity of the *I*(s) and the *non-I*(s).

Human(e) Bodies

The strength of the matrixial psychoanalysis lies in the possibility to conceive of the body outside the essentialist or biological frame and yet to provide it with certain proto-ethical qualities. The result of such an intervention is the proposition of a relation between corporeality and ethics that does not essentialize femininity and motherhood but nevertheless relies on certain prenatal/prematernal encounter-events that all the human beings have gone through and by which they have been non-consciously affected. The aim of this chapter has been to trace this relation in the dialogue between Emmanuel Lévinas and Bracha L. Ettinger, and in Ettinger's artistic works sharing her *Eurydice* trope. I have begun with establishing the linkage between the feminine body and the womb, claiming that the placement of the latter in the former allows us to make certain assumptions about the body. In an endeavor to portray the body as a prototype for connectedness and a primary site of the transsubjective, beyond historical encounter, I have turned to Emmanuel Lévinas's take on the body—including sensibility, the Moses figure, maternal corporeality, and the Other—and Ettinger's response to it. The tropes of the body, encounter, and connectedness beyond historical knowledge have returned in the section dealing with Ettinger's artistic practice. All these reflections contribute to the theorization of the feminine/motherly body as a site of the emergence and a dwelling-space of ethics: as a space of our human(e) origins.

Notes

1. Yet, one should not read the matrixial feminine as accessed by women exclusively. The matrixial feminine is, instead, non-Oedipal, non-phallic, and non-gendering as it is not reigned by the presence/absence paradigm. As a result, in Brian Massumi's words, "it is accessible to any body—on the condition that it surrenders itself to the several" (2006, 212).

2. The issue of corporeality also appears in Lévinas's theorization of the *face*; however, as I believe, this aspect is not vital for the argument presented in this chapter.

3. The excerpt Guenther analyzes in detail goes: "In proximity the absolutely other, the stranger whom I have 'neither conceived nor given birth to,' I already have on my arms, already bear, according to the Biblical formula, 'in my breast as the nurse bears the nurseling.' He has no other place, is not autochthonous, is uprooted, without a country, not an inhabitant, exposed to the cold and the heat of the seasons. To be reduced to having recourse to me is the homelessness or strangeness of the neighbor. It is incumbent on me" (Lévinas 1991, 91). The quotations used are from Numbers, XI, 12.

4. The issue of feminine otherness reappears in Lévinas's work. For instance, in *Time and the Other*, the woman becomes "essentially other" (Lévinas 1987, 86).

5. The notions of "side-by-sideness" and "besideness" return in Ettinger's descriptions of the matrixial stratum, usually describing the relation between the matrixial subjectivising sphere and phallic subjectivisation. They are also used in reference to the artistic encounter (see Ettinger 2011, 27).

6. Ettinger, *Eurydice*, No. 17, 1994–1996, oil, xerography with photocopic dust, pigment, and ashes on paper mounted on canvas, 26 x 52 cm, in Zegher and Pollock (2012, 82).

7. Although changes in Ettinger's *Eurydice* series do not always occur linearly, one can observe a certain tendency in Ettinger's late paintings, in which the women become increasingly indiscernible. See, for instance, *Eurydice*, No. 45, 2002–2006, oil on paper mounted on canvas, 24.2 x 29.7 cm, in Zegher and Pollock (2012, 168), and *Eurydice*, No. 50, 2006–2007, oil on paper mounted on canvas, 25.3 x 31.1 cm, in Zegher and Pollock (2012, 175).

8. Ettinger, *Eurydice*, No. 37, 2001, oil, xerography with photocopic dust, pigment, and ashes on paper mounted on canvas, 28.3 x 21.4 cm, in Zegher and Pollock (2012, 154).

9. Ettinger, *No Title-Sketch*, 1988–1989, xerography with photocopic dust, pigment, and ashes on paper, 22.3 x 24.9 cm, in Zegher and Pollock (2012, 207).

10. Ettinger, *No Title-Sketch*, 1985, xerography with photocopic dust, pigment, and ashes on paper, 27.3 x 23.1 cm, in Zegher and Pollock (2012, 203).

References

Barthes, Roland. 1981. *Camera Lucida: Reflections on Photography.* Translated by Richard Howard. New York: Hill and Wang.

Bevis, Kathryn. 2007. "'Better Than Metaphors'? Dwelling and the Maternal Body in Emmanuel Levinas." *Literature & Theology* 21 (3): 317–329.

Ettinger, Bracha L. 1993. *Matrix Halal(a)-Lapsus: Notes on Painting.* Oxford: Museum of Modern Art.

Ettinger, Bracha L. 2006a. "*Fascinance* and the Girl-to-m/Other Matrixial Feminine Difference." In *Psychoanalysis and the Image: Transdisciplinary Perspectives*, edited by Griselda Pollock, 60–93. Oxford: Blackwell Publishing Ltd.

Ettinger, Bracha L. 2006b. "The With-In-Visible Screen." In Bracha L. Ettinger, *The Matrixial Borderspace*, edited by Brian Massumi, 93–120. Minneapolis: University of Minnesota Press.

Ettinger, Bracha L. 2006c. "Weaving a Woman Artist with-in the Matrixial Encounter-Event." In Bracha L. Ettinger, *The Matrixial Borderspace*, edited by Brian Massumi, 173–198. Minneapolis: University of Minnesota Press.

Ettinger, Bracha L. 2006d. "Wit(h)nessing Trauma and the Matrixial Gaze." In Bracha L. Ettinger, *The Matrixial Borderspace*, edited by Brian Massumi, 123–155. Minneapolis: University of Minnesota Press.

Ettinger, Bracha L. 2011. "Uncanny Awe, Uncanny Compassion and Matrixial Transjectivity beyond Uncanny Anxiety." *French Literature Series* 38: 1–30.

Guenther, Lisa. 2006. "'Like a Maternal Body': Emmanuel Levinas and the Motherhood of Moses." *Hypatia* 21 (1): 119–136.

Lévinas, Emmanuel. 1969. *Totality and Infinity: An Essay on Exteriority.* Translated by Alphonso Lingis. Pittsburgh: Duquesne University Press.

Lévinas, Emmanuel. 1978. *Existence and Existents.* Translated by Alphonso Lingis. The Hague: Martinus Nijhoff.

Lévinas, Emmanuel. 1987. *Time and the Other (And Additional Essays).* Translated by Richard A. Cohen. Pittsburgh: Duquesne University Press.

Lévinas, Emmanuel. 1991. *Otherwise Than Being or Beyond Essence.* Translated by Alphonso Lingis. Dordrecht: Kluwer Academic Publishers.

Lévinas, Emmanuel. 2003. *On Escape. De l'évasion.* Translated by Bettina Bergo. Stanford: Stanford University Press.

Lévinas, Emmanuel, in conversation with Bracha L. Ettinger. 2006. "What Would Eurydice Say?" Translated by Joseph Simas and Carolyne Ducker. *Athena: Philosophical Studies* 2: 137–145.

Massumi, Brian. 2006. "Afterword. Painting: The Voice of the Grain." In Bracha L. Ettinger, *The Matrixial Borderspace*, edited by Brian Massumi, 201–213. Minneapolis: University of Minnesota Press.

Sontag, Susan. 1979. *On Photography.* London: Penguin Books.

Zegher, Catherine de, and Griselda Pollock, eds. 2012. *Art as Compassion: Bracha L. Ettinger.* Brussels: ASA Publishers.

11 The King's Four Bodies
Kantorowicz, Schmitt, Henry, and Hal

David Schauffler

The exposition of the "king's two bodies" that Ernst Kantorowicz offered in his 1957 work of that name has, since its appearance, provided a template for historical examination of medieval and Renaissance theories of political legitimacy and indeed for discussions of sovereignty in general. Depending on the emphasis one places on—or reads into—the constituent terms and the many medieval and early modern commentaries on their relation that Kantorowicz cites, the theory can be seen as leading toward either a constitutional or an authoritarian form of kingship—or, in historical terms, toward the parliamentary monarchy that developed in England or the absolutist form that came to prevail on the continent. To prefigure the following argument in brief: if an interpreter chooses to conflate the powers and the existences of the natural and symbolic bodies of the king, an authoritarian model will tend to result; if one sees these respective powers and *entia* as being different in kind, the scheme will predict a more constitutional structure.

The inherent ambiguity about the form of government evoked by the distinction between the king's natural and symbolic bodies allows us to use this distinction to comment on a specific issue that has not lost political relevance at the present day. This is the issue of succession of power, and in order to highlight it, we shall look at the seminal publication of the conservative, later Nazi, jurist Carl Schmitt, *Political Theology* (1922), and also at the incarnations and permutations of the king's "bodies" in Shakespeare's second Henrician tetralogy, specifically in *Richard II* and *Henry IV Parts 1 and 2*.[1] In the former we find a trenchant case made (though not in Kantorowicz's own language, obviously) for the perfect union of the natural body of the king with the symbolic body—a "sovereign" in which the executive function holds complete primacy over the legal, which depends upon it (Schmitt 2005, 28)—while in the latter, a much more fraught, even traumatic, relationship between symbolic and natural kingship is played out, against (as I shall argue) the background of an authorial conviction that the two, though necessarily combined in the person of the sovereign, are essentially separate and indeed opposed, and that the symbolic body of the king is not, in effect, a theological figure but a constitutional one.[2]

On the long list of dichotomies that can be attached to the pairing of the natural and symbolic bodies of the king, which include those of the person of the monarch and the institution of the crown, the executor of the laws and the legitimacy of the law (Kantorowicz 2016, chapter IV), and the physical incarnation of authority and its symbolic appurtenances or aura (e.g., Kantorowicz 2016, 336–338), prominent—and even, I would like to suggest, preeminent—is the dichotomy between the truncated reign of the natural king and the enduring reign of the symbolic king. In Kantorowicz this issue receives considerable attention, and he adduces much evidence testifying how great a concern it was to the jurists, chroniclers, and divines upon whom his argument draws. But he frames the issue in such a way as to obscure, I believe, the signal quality of the issue and its fundamental role in shaping the relation between the king's two bodies.

The issue is discussed at length in the long chapter of *The King's Two Bodies* entitled "The King Never Dies," which begins with the following adumbration:

> By interpreting the people as an *universitas* 'which never dies' the jurisprudents had arrived at the concept of a perpetuity of both the whole body politic (head and members together) and the constituent members alone. The perpetuity, however, of the 'head' alone was of equally great importance, since the head would usually appear as the responsible part and its absence might render the body corporate incomplete or incapable of action. The perpetuation of the head, therefore, created a new set of problems and led to new fictions.
>
> (Kantorowicz 2016, 314)

But this discussion, as the foregoing passage hints, is devoted largely to the symbolic dimension of royal succession—symbolism, to be fair, is the focus of Kantorowicz's work—and the connection between the continuity of government (represented by the king's immaterial, eternal body) and the prerogatives of government (represented by the king's material, executive body) is not directly addressed. "Not by any special act or decree," writes Kantorowicz of the establishment of dynastic primogeniture, "but *de facto*, both France in 1270 and England in 1272 recognized that the succession to the throne was the birthright of the eldest son: on the death—or burial—of the ruling monarch the son or legitimate heir became king automatically. . . . Henceforth, the king's true legitimation was dynastical, independent of approval or consecration on the part of the Church and independent also of election by the people" (2016, 330). For our purposes, it should be noted that Kantorowicz, following most of his sources, implicitly contrasts automatic dynastic succession with other "legitimating" succession strategies, namely consecration and election. This gives the impression—which may be correct—that the principal concern of thirteenth-century jurists was the form that succession was to take and not the fact of continuity in government (and government's prerogatives) itself, which, given the existence of the "king's eternal body" symbolism, may in some juridical discussions have been taken for granted.[3]

That this assumption was overly sanguine can easily be seen, for example, in the history of dynastic conflict that rocked England in the fifteenth century and France in the sixteenth, but a direct, and admirably succinct, constitutional assault on it can be found in the aforementioned monograph of Carl Schmitt. Schmitt was addressing different political circumstances than were Kantorowicz and his sources—namely, the incipient crisis of a constitutional democracy when what Habermas (1975) was to call "steering problems" result in a need for extrajudicial intervention in the practice of government—but his analysis of this situation very clearly outlines one essential feature of the relation between the king's "two bodies."

Political Theology famously begins with the announcement, "Sovereign is he who decides on the exception" (Schmitt 2005, 5), and the work consists essentially of a defense, or elucidation, of this proposal. The burden of the argument is that the sovereign—be it an individual in office, an individual in some other capacity, or a corporate body—is, by definition, that (or "he") which has the power of decision; specifically, the power to decide when the rule of law must be suspended (Schmitt 2005, 6–8). Note that the sovereign, according to Schmitt, is not that (or he) which simply executes extrajudicial action once the exception has been declared or otherwise found to exist. It is, rather, the organ that identifies, or declares, the exception itself; the organ, in other words, that determines the limit of operation of the rule of law.

This is, initially, a plausible definition of sovereignty, especially if we assume (as Schmitt appears to do)[4] that if the power to suspend the rule of law is not held by one entity, it will of necessity be held by another, making that other entity, perforce, the "sovereign." This is a tautology characteristic of Schmitt's argumentation throughout, in which assumptions are made about the nature of the political constitution that are found to necessitate a conclusion linked to them by logic. The most fundamental of these assumptions, and the one that drives the rest, is that no constitutional order is capable of anticipating all the conflicts that arise within a society or dangers that impend from without, so that, inevitably, every constitutional order will be confronted sooner or later with "the exception," at which point the question of sovereignty, which may rest implicit up to that point, will become, so to speak, activated:

> It is precisely the exception that makes relevant the subject of sovereignty, that is, the whole question of sovereignty. The precise details of the emergency cannot be anticipated, nor can one spell out what

may take place in such a case, especially when it is truly a matter of an extreme emergency and of how it is to be eliminated. . . . The most guidance the constitution can provide is to indicate who can act in such a case. If such action is not subject to controls, if it is not hampered in some way by checks and balances, as is the case in a liberal constitution, then it is clear who the sovereign is. He decides whether there is an extreme emergency as well as what must be done to eliminate it.

(Schmitt 2005, 6–7)

The exception, which has been introduced as the moment in which the question of sovereignty becomes acute, is here revealed as, rather, a tool of sovereignty, that is, as a characteristic or power inherent to the sovereign and indeed definitive of his sovereignty. And crucial to this understanding of sovereignty is its volitional quality: Schmitt castigates his liberal counterparts for "objectivism" (see Schmitt 2005, 28–29) and argues that the executive is by nature a subjective function: "the conception of personality and its connection with formal authority arose from a specific juristic interest, namely, an especially clear awareness of what the legal decision entails" (2005, 30). The entailment is, according to him, precisely the maxim of interpretation, such that it is the essence of the judge to weigh and sift the facts of the case rather than, for example, simply hand down a mandatory sentence; it is the essence of the parliamentarian to filter the demands of her constituents rather than reflect them immediately as if by referendum; and likewise it is the essence of the sovereign to act personally rather than mechanically.

In support of his claim that the sovereign's power to declare the exception—to abrogate the constitution—is inherent, Schmitt turns to the sixteenth-century jurist and political theorist Jean Bodin, specifically the section of Bodin's *Republic* in which he argues that the prince ceases to be bound to his duty to the people "under conditions of urgent necessity" (Schmitt 2005, 8). But at the same time Schmitt blithely dismisses Bodin's most famous formulation, which will return us to the question of the king's two bodies, namely, "sovereignty is the absolute and perpetual power of a republic" (quoted in Schmitt 2005, 8).

It is precisely the perpetuity of sovereignty that most tellingly expounds the character of the king's two bodies and that at the same time most forcefully, in my view, indicts Schmitt's posit that the sovereign is he who declares the exception. In regard to the first, I have mentioned above that it forms a crucial concern of Kantorowicz and the jurists whose views he considers; obviously, in a monarchial form of government, the mortal span of the natural king—be he sovereign or some more limited kind of executive—forecasts and demands both a form of succession that will guarantee continuity of government and also an ideological device that will confer continuity of legitimacy as well. Schmitt, in contrast, appears curiously insensitive to the issue of continuity and to the very grave implications it has for his theory of sovereignty. It is possible that he assumed that under a constitutional framework in which the sovereign was elected or appointed to office, the same protocols by which this came about would simply survive—indeed, along with the entire constitution—the "extreme emergency" which the sovereign declares and by which he asserts his sovereignty, but there are no grounds for this assumption; indeed, it could be imagined that the most delectable "exception" a sovereign could possibly decide on would be precisely the exception to a constitutional limit on his term in office. In any event, if the sovereign is, as Schmitt has it, in essence the adjudicator of the rule of law, then we are effectively dealing with a case parallel to that of monarchy, where the death or abdication of the sovereign demands a procedure for the transfer both of executive power and of legitimacy.

The exception cited by Schmitt as the breach or suspension of constitutional order and, therefore, as the proof and revelation of the sovereign, is described by him, as we have seen above, as essentially indescribable: this is presented as being due to the contingent nature of the circumstances, but it is more exactly because it is, according to Schmitt, the prerogative of the sovereign to "decide on" the exception and he can, "if not hampered in some way by checks and balances," decide that the exception is anything at all. However, for purposes of discussion it may be helpful to try to specify further what, under a monarchial or other form of absolutist sovereignty, might be considered an exception in the way Schmitt introduces it, that is, a crisis of governance in which the constitutional order, confronted with a situation for which it has no remedy, must be suspended.

In *Legitimation Crisis* (1973), Jürgen Habermas analyzes this situation less obliquely than Schmitt, and his analysis may yield some concepts helpful for looking at the relation between the king's two bodies. Citing systems theory, Habermas writes that "crises arise when the structure of a social system allows fewer possibilities for problem-solving than are necessary to the continued existence of the system" (1975, 2). That is to say (setting aside the details of Habermas's argument), a crisis occurs when the system—organism, community, or polity—produces problems that are not soluble under the existing protocols possessed by that system. So far this looks rather like Schmitt's "exception," namely the emergency that requires suspension of the constitutional order for the very purpose (we may assume) of saving it. But it is soon clear that in Habermas's analysis the stress has crucially shifted; the system is construed organically—as was, both figuratively and literally, the medieval realm—and thus as possessing an inherent identity, and it is this identity that the constitutional order both reflects and preserves. So the crisis that afflicts the constitutional order is not a crisis of that order as such (though it may take this shape), but a crisis of the competence of that order, and the sovereign remedy can only be that which restores the competence of the constitutional order to reflect and preserve the system, or the polity.

This construal of the crisis, or exception, emphatically replaces the subjectivity that Schmitt was so careful to reserve to the executive, and thus to the sovereign, in the polity itself (however that, in turn, is to be framed).[5] If the political community is held to be in any sense organic, and if the constitutional order (and thus the crisis in or exception to that order, and therefore, in Schmitt's terms, the expression or exercise of sovereignty) is conceived as a means of preserving and perpetuating that organism, then it is only the political organism, the polity, that can apprehend and declare the crisis, that can, as Schmitt would have it, "make the decision" (2005, 6). Habermas is explicit on this point: "Systems are not presented as subjects; but . . . only subjects can be involved in crises. Thus, *only* when members of a society experience structural alterations as critical for continued existence and feel their social identity threatened can we speak of crises. . . . Crisis states assume the form of the disintegration of social institutions" (1975, 3). In this reading it is above all the sovereign (however constituted) that cannot decide on the exception; the exception is precisely the moment in which sovereign power (whether conceived as superordinate to the constitutional order or as that order itself) fails in its office.

Failure in office is a condition that can be diagnosed only under circumstances in which the office and its holder are clearly distinguishable, which brings us back to the relation of the body natural and body political of the king. As mentioned at the outset, the second Henrician tetralogy of Shakespeare gives us an apt opportunity for examining this relation in several permutations, and in the course of so doing we may perhaps further be able to clarify the implications of the competing theories of sovereign power and crisis of Schmitt and Habermas discussed above.

In *The King's Two Bodies*, Kantorowicz famously includes an analysis of *Richard II*, which, he says, "is the tragedy of the King's Two Bodies" (2016, 26). This is clearly intended to emphasize that the character of Richard II incarnates the ambiguity of the symbolic formulation: he takes himself to be, at the same time and in the same degree, both the body natural and the body politic of the king. That this is a mistake, a category error, is evident in the narrative arc of the play and is emphasized by Kantorowicz in his reading of it; he looks closely at the language of three central scenes, writing, "in each one of these three scenes we encounter the same cascading from divine kingship to kingship's 'Name,' and from the name to the naked misery of man" (2016, 27). We need not here recapitulate Kantorowicz's discussion of these scenes, which is, in any case, more particularly devoted to Richard's psychological transformation than to his political convictions, but it is abundantly evident from the text of the play that Richard's sin has been to conflate the natural body with the body politic and to assume to his person the majesty that pertains to the office. In one of the play's most famous speeches, he admonishes his companions that a man and a king are two different kinds of being:

> Throw away respect,
> Tradition, form, and ceremonious duty;
> For you have but mistook me all this while.
> I live with bread, like you; feel want,
> Taste grief, need friends. Subjected thus,
> How can you say to me I am a king?
>   (*Richard II*, Act III, sc. 2, 172–177)

It is the sign of Richard's own continued megalomania that he believes that a king cannot be subjected to natural human constraints and that if he is, he cannot be a king. The position, making allowances for difference in tone, is exactly analogous to Carl Schmitt's thesis that the sovereign cannot be "hampered in some way by checks and balances" and if he is, he is not the sovereign. The complete identification of office and man, of symbolic body and natural body, appears in *Richard II* as a clear psychological problem, but it is also just as clearly a political one: Richard's downfall comes about, briefly, because of his whimsical and arbitrary rule; he governs "without checks and balances" and continually asserts that it is his prerogative to do so. But the specific causal factor that leads to Bolingbroke's return and Richard's swift collapse has to do with, as I have mentioned earlier, what might be considered the crux of the issue of sovereign authority: the question of succession. Immediately upon the death of John of Gaunt, Richard determines to seize his holdings, thus disinheriting Bolingbroke (Duke of Hereford), the rightful heir. Richard's uncle, the Duke of York, protests in language that reveals the theoretical import of this action:

> Take Hereford's rights away, and take from Time
> His charters and his customary rights.
> Let not tomorrow then ensue today.
> Be not thyself; for how art thou a king
> But by fair sequence and succession?
>   (*Richard II*, Act II, sc. 1, 190–199)

Richard, deeming himself to *be* the law, believes that he can "decide on the exception" at will; he neglects to see that he is sovereign only because of the law; that if he, in Habermas's terms, brings about the disintegration of social institutions (such as property and inheritance rights), he, in effect, disinherits himself of office.

The situation is quite different in the two Henry IV plays; here, conveniently enough, we have two characters who may be said to represent, in partial ways, the two aspects of the king's two bodies. When *Henry*

IV Part 1 opens, Henry has already been on the throne long enough to become shaken and "wan with care" (*Henry IV Part 1*, Act I, sc. 1, 1) and it is clear that young Prince Hal will not wait much longer before inheriting the throne (if indeed he and his father are not deposed in one of what is portrayed as a succession of rebellions, active and incipient). We are therefore presented with a holder of the kingly office (albeit through usurpation) and a natural man who has leisure to contemplate precisely the difference between himself as a man and himself in his (future) capacity as king; it would not be a gross oversimplification to say that the nature of this difference is the main thematic object of the *Henry IV* plays.

In light of our earlier suggestion that succession of authority is the test case of the limit of sovereign power and of its relation to the constitutional order, let it be noted that King Henry, whom as I have said we might provisionally identify with the body politic, the symbolic kingly body, is as a character occupied in both the *Henry IV* plays almost exclusively with the issue of succession and peaceful transfer of power: first, in the suppression of rebellion and second, in the apparently debauched habits of his heir, Prince Hal. In regard to the first, it is repeated both in the plays and in criticism that Henry's tumultuous reign is by way of expiation for the sin of usurpation: he has overturned the constitutional order by taking power and his reign is consumed, therefore, with what is in effect the restoration (and preservation) of the constitutional order. However, it has been said above that most readings of *Richard II* would see Richard as the author of his own downfall, on grounds of defect of character or abuse of office or, in Habermas's terms, the generation of crisis.[6] And thus the work of restoration of the constitutional order is, on Henry's part, notably impersonal; indeed, our inclination to see him as in some way representing the king's "body politic" is abetted by what seems to be a complete devotion to office. He appears, night and day, beset by worries and preoccupied with governance, and the word that accompanies him from the first line of *Henry IV Part 1* to the last act of *Henry IV Part 2* is "care." Here there is no hint of an "identification" of the natural body with the symbolic body; rather, the former simply suffers under the burden of the latter.

It is Prince Hal who exhibits, on our reading, the most evident awareness of the "king's two bodies" and some conscious reflection on the relation between them. His inheritance of his father's crown will, when it comes, reestablish the constitutional order at its most sensitive point, and the confusion that occurs in Act IV, sc. 5 when Hal, thinking the king dead, takes the crown, emphasizes the fragility of the moment of succession—the juxtaposition of the mortal and the immortal elements of sovereignty. In the same scene, Henry tells his son "thou seek'st the greatness that will overwhelm thee" (*Henry IV Part 2*, Act IV, sc. 5, 97) but Hal has by this time fully weighed the articulation of the king's two bodies and it seems evident that he will be overwhelmed neither by megalomania, like Richard, nor by "care," like his father.

It is in the father-son relationship (which is, as has frequently been pointed out, complicated by Hal's friendship with Falstaff and in *Henry IV Part 1* by King Henry's admiration for Hotspur) that the question both of kingship as such and of royal succession—of the continuity of the sovereign power—is most prominently examined. The disobedience of Prince Hal as a son parallels the political disobedience of the rebels, but there is a crucial difference: Prince Hal views his father *qua* father but also *qua* king; that is, he sees him in the first instance as the body natural, toward whom rebellion and misbehavior are comparatively trivial, natural, and forgivable offenses but yet again as the body politic, the symbolic body, to whom, as the embodiment of the polity, ultimate loyalty and obedience are due (and of course, Hal's resolution to throw off his bad courses and low friends upon succession to the crown are the token of this ultimate obedience). Hal's quasi-filial relation to Falstaff, while not at all obedient, is more affectionate, inclining us still further to think that emotionally he, too, sees King Henry principally in the role of king, and this inclination takes further force from the fact that Hal's emotional, or, so to say, filial, reconciliation with his father in the deathbed scene takes place more or less at the same time as his final repudiation of Falstaff. King Henry, for his part, likewise splits his paternal feelings along the lines of the king's two bodies: he plays toward Hal the role of the frustrated and then forgiving father, the natural man; for Hotspur, though this theme is raised only in passing, as it were, he feels admiration and envies Northumberland for being the father of "a son who is the theme of honor's tongue" (*Henry IV Part 1*, Act I, sc. 1, 80)—that is, precisely a son who would be a suitable successor to the crown and who would perpetuate, as Kantorowicz has it, the *dignitas non moritur*. The rebels, unlike Hal, deny King Henry the dignity of the symbolic body, for having aided him in his usurpation they continue to see him as a usurper; that is, as one who holds the crown as a natural man but has not the *dignitas* of the office and is not owed the allegiance due to it. Shakespeare does not pronounce on the justness of their view but gives a clear opinion on the rightness of it; it is wrong because it perpetuates civil strife and resists the restoration of the constitutional order. And, in the character of Hotspur, in *Henry IV Part 1*, there are clear tokens that King Henry is wrong in his assessment; Hotspur evinces traits of character—arrogance, stubbornness, willfulness, and pique—that recall with some exactness the failings of Richard II and imply that Hotspur, were he to become the sovereign, would fail in the role as Richard had done and for the same reason, namely, for conflating the king's two bodies entirely and assuming, as Schmitt was to do, that the natural body could completely absorb the body politic and decide the exception.

The constitutional lesson of the three plays discussed is, I believe, fairly legible, if we consider it in the vocabulary we have adopted from Kantorowicz, Schmitt, and Habermas. The king as sovereign can indeed be said to have two bodies, or to embody two principles: one—the symbolic body, the body politic, the eternal body—is assumed by the king upon his coronation and confers upon him the executive power wielded by the other body: the natural body, the spatial and temporal body, the mortal body, and, to echo Schmitt, the subjective body. The sovereign is the second, but the sovereign power is in the first; and the rule of good monarchizing is to remain alive to the distinction. Schmitt is correct to hold that the executive (as do other orders of constitutional authority) contains a crucial moment of subjectivity, but to deduce from this an essential autonomy of sovereign authority is to create anarchy at the core of sovereignty itself. As York cautioned Richard, capriciousness in execution of power delegitimizes the executive, for it undercuts the relation of the symbolic body to the natural one or, as we might put it, deprecates the constitutional order according to which the sovereign takes authority. This delegitimation does indeed produce the "exception," but it is not, as Schmitt would have it, the sovereign's prerogative; it is, rather, his failure, and it is "decided" not by the sovereign but by the polity. The repair of the exception, of the crisis, comes about, as Habermas suggests, not through extrajudicial executive action, but through restoring or improving the "steering mechanism" (1975, 7) of the constitutional order. In response to the crisis of Richard's arbitrary rule and his own usurpation of the crown, Henry IV is caught in a ten-year "legitimation crisis" that he can only quell by rigorous "objectification" of his role, subsumption of the natural body in the body politic (rather than, as with Richard, the other way round), and as a result he finds kingship a crushing burden; nor is his reign, except negatively, a success. But Prince Hal, having weighed the relation of subjectivity to authority, of the body natural to the body politic, and of the temporal to the perpetual, is prepared for his reign; he can assume the authority of the crown, without assuming that the authority is his own, by keeping the distinction between the king's two bodies clear to himself and others. Upon his father's death, being greeted by the Chief Justice as "Your Majesty," he replies, "This new and gorgeous garment, majesty,/Sits not so easy on me as you think" (*Henry IV Part 2*, Act 5, sc. 2, 44–46).

Notes

1. This selection of sources leads to unavoidable anachronism in certain respects of their comparison; my hope is that at the level of generality appropriate to a chapter of short length, such anachronism need not impede the argument.
2. Because the focus of this chapter is upon the restricted issue of succession of power, I will not address the question of the relations of politics to theology, which relations occupy a prominent part in the sources I am drawing upon.

3. The same impression—that is, of greater concern being devoted to the manner of succession than to its constitutional significance—persists through the first half of Kantorowicz's exhaustive discussion of contemporary sources, namely, until he begins to discuss the "third notion" of *dignitas*, which he honestly, but not very helpfully, partially conflates with *officium regis*. See Kantorowicz (2016, 314–382) and discussion below.
4. In his Introduction to the cited edition of *Political Theology*, George Schwab includes a brief contextualization, or apologium, for Schmitt's argument in which he stresses the latter's fear of threats to constitutional order arising both within (anti-constitutional parties) and without (putschists), characterizing Schmitt's conception of sovereignty as an effort "to save the Weimar state" from such dangers. See Schmitt (2005, xli–xlix).
5. It is not part of the argument of this chapter to dispute the constitution of the polity, or the estates, in Jean Bodin's terms: we are simply taking for granted a constituency which, however it is comprised, makes up the political community over which the sovereign and constitutional order have effective authority. For present purposes the question is not how that political community is constituted, but what relation of duty it has to the organs under discussion, namely the sovereign and the constitutional order.
6. Habermas makes an interesting point, which cannot be pursued further here, that ideological and symbolic factors become more prominent the greater the integrative failings of the system and the more, therefore, the system loses legitimacy. As Richard II succumbs to rebellion and defeatism, his preoccupation with the symbolic elements of kingship grows ever greater. The same direct association between incompetence and venality in governing and the language of honor, patriotism, and traditional values can be observed in certain contemporary societies.

References

Habermas, Jürgen. 1975. *Legitimation Crisis*. Translated by Thomas McCarthy. Boston: Beacon Press.

Kantorowicz, Ernst H. 2016. *The King's Two Bodies: A Study in Medieval Political Theology*. Princeton: Princeton University Press.

Schmitt, Carl. 2005. *Political Theology: Four Chapters on the Concept of Sovereignty*. Translated by George Schwab. Chicago, IL: University of Chicago Press.

Shakespeare, William. "*Henry IV, Part One* from Folger Digital Texts." In *Folger Shakespeare Library*, edited by Barbara Mowat, Paul Werstine, Michael Poston, and Rebecca Niles. Accessed on October 30, 2018. www.folgerdigitaltexts.org

Shakespeare, William. "*Henry IV, Part Two* from Folger Digital Texts." In *Folger Shakespeare Library*, edited by Barbara Mowat, Paul Werstine, Michael Poston, and Rebecca Niles. Accessed on October 30, 2018. www.folgerdigitaltexts.org

Shakespeare, William. "*Richard II* from Folger Digital Texts." In *Folger Shakespeare Library*, edited by Barbara Mowat, Paul Werstine, Michael Poston, and Rebecca Niles. Accessed on October 30, 2018. www.folgerdigitaltexts.org

Contributors

Steffan Blayney is a Research Fellow in the Department of History at the University of Sheffield, UK. His research focuses on the relations between health, the body and society, and on histories of activism. He is a co-founder and organizer of History Acts, a workshop and network connecting historians and activists.

Carlo Bovolo is now collaborating with the Museum of Criminal Anthropology "Cesare Lombroso" of the University of Turin (Italy). In 2017 he gained a PhD in History at the University of Eastern Piedmont (Italy) and, in the same year, he was a fellow of the Fondazione Filippo Burzio (Turin, Italy).

Christopher E. Forth is the Dean's Professor of Humanities and Professor of History at the University of Kansas, USA. His books include *Zarathustra in Paris* (2001), *The Dreyfus Affair and the Crisis of French Manhood* (2004), *Masculinity in the Modern West* (2008), and *Fat: A Cultural History of the Stuff of Life* (2019).

Kylo-Patrick R. Hart is the Chair of the Department of Film, Television, and Digital Media at Texas Christian University, USA, where he teaches courses in film and television history, theory, and criticism; popular culture; and queer media studies. He is the author or editor of several books about media.

Jacqueline Susann Holler is an Associate Professor of History and Coordinator of Women's and Gender Studies at the University of Northern British Columbia in Prince George, Canada. She is author of *Escogidas Plantas: Nuns and Beatas in Mexico City, 1531–1601*, of texts in Latin American history and gender studies, and of articles and chapters on early colonial Mexican history.

Justyna Jajszczok is an Assistant Professor at the Institute of English, University of Silesia, Katowice, Poland. She has co-edited four collections of essays and published articles on nineteenth-century literature and culture. Her research interests include Victorian science and literature, history of life sciences, and invasion literature.

Anna Kisiel is a PhD student in Literary Studies at the University of Silesia in Katowice, Poland. Her research revolves around matrixial psycho-analysis, trauma studies, photography theory, and body and femininity in the visual arts and literature. Currently she is working on her dissertation concerning the body in Ettinger's theory and art.

Claude Lacroix is an Associate Professor and Chairperson of the Art History and Theory Program at Bishop's University, Canada. He holds a PhD from the École des Hautes Études en Sciences Sociales, Paris. His research focuses on the representation of the body and gender, body fluids in artworks, and public art.

William Leeming is an Associate Professor at OCAD University, Toronto, Canada, lecturing in a range of subject areas including the social sciences and science and technology studies. His research of the last 20 years has focused on the history of technology adoption in science and technology.

Aleksandra Musiał is an Assistant Professor at the Institute of English Cultures and Literatures, University of Silesia, Katowice, Poland. She has written about, among other subjects, representations of the war in Vietnam. Her research interests include American history and culture, and the intersections of history, ideology, and myth.

Willemijn Ruberg is an Associate Professor in Cultural History at Utrecht University, the Netherlands. Her research interests include the history of the body, gender, and forensic science. She is leading the research project "Forensic Culture. A Comparative Analysis of Forensic Practices in Europe, 1930–2000," funded by an ERC Consolidator Grant.

David Schauffler studied at Oberlin College and New York University, USA, and Nicolaus Copernicus University in Toruń, Poland, from which he received a PhD in Philosophy. He teaches in the Department of English at the University of Silesia in Katowice, Poland, concentrating upon American nineteenth-century literature and nineteenth- and twentieth-century social philosophy.

CalvinJohn Smiley, PhD, is an Assistant Professor in the Sociology Department of Hunter College-CUNY, USA. His research focuses on issues of race, punishment, and social justice. More specifically, he has done research on issues of reentry in the United States for individuals exiting prison settings.

Index